The Magic in Your Hands

BRIAN SNELLGROVE

THE MAGIC
IN YOUR HANDS

HOW TO SEE AURAS
AND USE THEM FOR DIAGNOSIS
AND HEALING

Illustrated by Kate Aldous
Index compiled by Mary Kirkness

SAFFRON WALDEN
THE C.W. DANIEL COMPANY LIMITED

First published in 1997 by Econ Verlag GmbH, Düsseldorf und München
under the title: *Das Geheimnis von Aura und Chakras*
This completely revised, illustrated English-language edition
first published in Great Britain in 1998
by The C.W. Daniel Company Limited
1 Church Path, Saffron Walden,
Essex, CB10 1JP, United Kingdom

ISBN 0 85207 315 1

The Random House Group Limited supports The Forest Stewardship
Council (FSC®), the leading international forest certification organisation.
Our books carrying the FSC label are printed on FSC® certified paper.
FSC is the only forest certification scheme endorsed by the leading
environmental organisations, including Greenpeace. Our
paper procurement policy can be found at
www.randomhouse.co.uk/environment

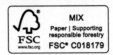

Printed and bound in Great Britain by Clays Ltd, St Ives PLC

Produced by
Book Production Consultants plc,
25–27 High Street, Chesterton, Cambridge CB4 1ND
Typeset by Cambridge Photosetting Services

Contents

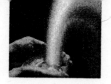

THE MYSTERY OF CREATION

We are surrounded by mysteries from a whole range of hidden or inexplicable phenomena. The word itself derives from the Greek word *muo*, closed lips or eyes. Bees are able to fly when conventional aerodynamic theory says that it is impossible. There is a theory that the earth is being visited by intelligent beings. The rocks in Death Valley, Utah, appear to move by themselves. People catch fire for no reason. Ghosts inhabit a particular room or a theatre. Some would even say that love itself is a mystery. Many scientists would define a mystery as simply that which has not yet been explained but given time will surely be. But whether it is the wind in the trees on a cold dark night, or speculation on the dark side of the moon, these mysteries produce an equal measure of fascination and fear among the general population.

History is full of events with no explanation. An old Scottish prayer seeks deliverance from "shadowy ghoulies and ghosties and long-legged beasties and things that go bump in the night". The English writer H. G. Wells encapsulated this mixture of curiosity and fear in an early novel set in Industrial England, creating the concept of the 'Invisible Man'. The idea of an interloper in our midst seeing everything while going completely unnoticed himself is a very evocative piece of phantasy. However, we all know that the story, although well constructed, is ultimately not plausible. Yet the phenomena of 'things that go bump in the night' has been reclassified as 'parapsychological phenomena' and receives considerable respect. At the same time many scientists dismiss or ignore phenomena that do not have a rational explanation, cannot be measured by scientific apparatus, or appear to happen beyond the confines of the cranium, reducing them to figments of the imagination or gullibility.

It is perhaps significant that the word 'mystery' does not occur in the old testament of the Bible. It is not until the new testament that we find eternal truths, and the significance of mysteries, signs and wonders unfolding. Some would say that the death and resurrection of Christ was one of the most mysterious events of all time. Do mysteries transgress the laws of nature, or is it that our understanding of the laws of the universe needs to be vastly expanded to grasp the possibilities?

In the face of events that are outside the range of our comprehension, are we being asked to suspend our reason and humbly accept that we are ignorant?

Or does our rational mind have a duty to de-mystify the mystery, to refuse to accept any phenomenon outside our knowledge until it is somehow tamed and brought into order? We will do ourselves a service if we view the topic of the aura with a dispassionate but kindly eye.

WHO ARE WE?

We can't help being curious about the nature of our existence. It's an instinct. We all know that we came from somewhere and we are going somewhere. We also instinctively attribute a sense of healing to where we are now, the intermediate realm of physical life. The idea that there are other levels of reality can be disorientating to our conscious mind, since it reveals our usual perception of the world to be limited.

Accepting the idea and influence of the aura – the interface between matter and spirit – requires a fundamental paradigm shift in our thinking. This shift has already happened in the world of physics as classical Newtonian physics was found to be too limited relative to modern physics. Classical physics described objects and the relationship between them as we experience them through our senses. These rules 'make sense' to us – a wooden table is simply a solid table. Modern physics by contrast shows that objects are made up of particles and waves and the space between them. Moreover, it reveals that what we see depends on our position at the time. The viewpoint of the observer influences what is seen – particle or wave. Though these observations are counter to our conventional grasp of nature they are generally accepted.

Whilst we may choose to ignore these important questions in the normal course of our life, we are inexorably drawn to them when we have a paranormal experience, when a loved one dies or when there is great danger. In an impending plane crash, or when a friend has had an accident and lies between life and death, we instinctively pray to God even if we would normally not admit to any beliefs. It is therefore both intelligent and wise to keep an open mind.

Primitive man was plunged by nature into a place where, like an animal, he behaved instinctively. Maintaining his territory was essential for preserving life and he was only aware of the problems of existence at a very basic level. Existence followed simple rules – protect yourself, eat enough and live, starve and die. Even at this early stage, he was using his powers of detection – via the aura – to ascertain the approach of dangerous animals. We would now call that quality 'instinct'.

Some stages later, in the early civilizations of Egypt and Sumeria, we find that man has an awareness of a whole, a pattern to life with meaning and purpose. However this was not to be achieved through his own effort but by mystical revelation from the gods. He believed that he had been created by God or the gods and it was his task to serve them. The Egyptian Pharaoh was regarded as a semi-god and through his authority, god-given civilization was shaped. Depicted in Egyptian art as far larger than ordinary men, the Pharaoh dispensed wisdom not of himself but as a channel for the gods. The same thing applied to the Sumerian priest-kings.

However in the course of time man became aware that he had to stand on his own two feet not only physically but spiritually. The Greeks began to be aware of themselves as physical beings. They glorified the body and, rejecting the wisdom of the gods and the demands of authority developed their own wisdom. While the Greeks applied their thinking to the religious concepts of the world, the Romans took up this thinking ability and applied it to the practical activities of everyday life, and thereby came about the Roman ego-man, a powerful individual who acts out of his own resources.

At that period Christianity arose, teaching that man should develop and use his personal resources for higher aims and purposes. The founder taught that serving humanity in general was more important than self-serving and self-regarding acts. He claimed to be the Son of God and showed "the way, the truth and the life". Religion through the ages has gone through phases of the capitulating human will to divine law. With the Renaissance ('rebirth') came the beginning of the freeing of the individual from dependence on tradition and reliance on his own potential in all walks of life – the arts, commerce, exploration, science. From this time on, Western man has increasingly developed and worked out of his own resources, as does the individual emerging from teenage into adulthood.

Our present society places great emphasis on the freedom to pursue one's own aims and goals. In so far as selfishness predominates, this is a reaching back to the territorial instincts of the cave person causing a diminution in the quality of the community.

In spite of the advance of technology there remains a hunger for 'something' with which to make sense not only of life but of death. Generally speaking the split between science and mysticism has not been healed. Rudolph Steiner in the last century attempted to apply scientific objectivity to mysticism. Currently, scientific interest in psi is also growing. PSI is short for psychic including the four phenomena – precognition, telepathy, clairvoyance and psychokinesis or PK.

A large volume of research data has accumulated, and it is becoming more difficult for sceptical scientists to avoid confrontations with their more adventurous colleagues. The unexplained findings in all sciences – previously cast aside in favour of more tangible investigation – are now being openly tackled, even by some scientists who once kept their psi research clandestine out of great fear for jobs and reputation. It is amazing how a recently retired scientist suddenly develops an interest in psi. The secret life of scientists would fill numerous volumes!

IS THERE A DIFFERENCE BETWEEN SPIRIT AND MATTER?

Logical positivism in general, and David Hume in particular, believes that nothing exists outside the physical, observed world. Any philosophical and religious systems are redundant in the face of the developments of modern science and technology. However, no matter which religion or philosophic system we consider (except materialism and atheism), each tells us that apart from our material world there exists a quantumly different and complimentary one – the world of Spirit. For Christians it is the Holy Spirit, for Hindus it is para-atman.

For most individuals, reconciling the world of spirit with the world of matter is a long journey, never satisfactorily resolved. Life is lived as a consumer, as a creature on a treadmill – essentially without thinking. Life is to be consumed, for what are we but consumers? However, we stand in danger of falling into a trap. With our physical senses, we see the world of things and possessions, food, entertainment, travel and all the things that make western civilization function. This comprises awesome materialism promoted by the corporate world and the mass media. It dictates a vast array of wants and hopes. Our practical life has become deeply rooted in this 'reality'. Exploring ways of alternative thinking has become extremely difficult. It requires an extraordinary act of will, self-examination and lack of fear to acknowledge that happiness does not equal the acquisition of goods in the market place.

Because our psychical senses and vistas have become blunted over the generations, we are not able to view the other world – the spiritual world – which is just as much a 'material' world as this more familiar physical world. The only difference is that the 'material' is of a different type. There is not a sudden change from one to the other, rather there are gradations of matter. For example the physical world is made up of solids, liquids, gasses and the ionic layer. The most unchanging or stable form is the physical. There are various other ethereal layers, each subject to their own particular laws. It may be helpful to see 'solid matter' as forming one end of a tube, and 'soul' as comprising the other. Between them are all the other states. If we are to understand life to the full, all types of 'matter' must be understood and entertained with equal respect.

'Material' is to do with the matter from which something is made – visible or invisible to the human eye is not the point. Matter in the spiritual universe is more subtle, more difficult to measure but just as vital. The laws in this spiritual world are quite different, but just as inexorable and reliable as Newton and the apple, or Archimedes and his famous theorem.

Aeons ago, for example in Egypt, an approach uniting science and religion would have been taken for granted and was the working model for everyday life. Astrologers and clairvoyants worked together with architects and army generals to advise the ruler.

WILL SCIENCE AND RELIGION EVER UNITE?

One of the problems with our modern society is that because of the abuse of power by the church, and the general misunderstanding of what constitutes religion, most people have rejected all that religion stands for. There have been great scientists and scientific thinkers who have, over the years, striven to create a united world view. Einstein was in the process of this when he died. In contrast, atheists have been few in number. Hence in the middle there is a gulf, a vacuum. In its place sits the god of profit and consumerism. Rainforests are pillaged. Society compromises its principles for immediate gain. Families break down. Violence increases.

Yet this is not found to be satisfactory at a deep level. Even with this disturbance we find signs of cooperation between mystics and scientists to rediscover more and more links and connections between these apparently contradictory worlds. Will it ever be 'scientific' to believe in God? One might ask if is it intelligent not to.

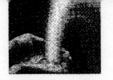

PART ONE

THE AURA

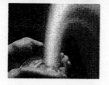

CHAPTER ONE

THE AURA – HISTORICAL OBSERVATIONS

Everything and everyone has an 'aura'. This word 'aura' comes from the Latin air, which in turn comes from the Greek word for breeze, or breath. It is not religious or spiritual though over the years it has been linked with spiritual qualities.

The notion of an aura or a light body coming from the human being is as old as history itself. This light was known in Hebrew as the Shekinah, or luminous Presence of God. Many examples are cited in the Bible including the dazzling light encountered by Moses at the burning bush, and on Mount Sinai when he descended with the tablets engraved with the Ten Commandments. The light shining around him was so bright that the children of Israel were unable to look upon it. An exceedingly brilliant light shone around St. Paul when he had his vision at the time of his conversion on the road to Damascus. It is reputed that when St. John of the Cross knelt at prayer at the altar, a 'certain brightness' darted from his face. St. Philip Neri was constantly seen enveloped in light.

The awareness of the aura has featured as long as civilized man has existed. Auras are mainly linked with the human being; plants and stones also radiate after a fashion, but because they cannot think in the way we understand it (as far as we know), their aura is more likely to be determined by the more predictable biological attributes.

The word 'aura' does not only mean the radiation that comes from each one of us, but it can also be used to mean the collective energy produced together by all of us in society, and that includes the whole planet. Everything that we all do – or don't do – plays its part in the integrity of that aura.

Living organisms, including man, are not only affected by light, but they emit light. The bioluminescence of bacteria, fire flies and deep sea fish has been known for centuries. The Russian biologist Alexander Gurvich observed that mitoses were stimulated at a point on an onion root when the tip of a second onion root was pointed at it. The roots were shielded from each other with glass (although the effect only occured if quartz glass, not ordinary glass, was used). It appeared that UV radiation was stimulating cell division acting on biological organisms and propagating 'secondary emissions'. He christened this phenomenon 'mitogenic radiation'. Such radiation increases during muscle contraction and where there is tumour tissue. Later in Russia, Professor Inyushin, at the Kazakh State University, Alma-Ata, postulated the main source of this mitogenic radiation was the nucleus of the cell.

Apart from these biological effects, there is also a 'cocktail' of electromagnetic field effects from radio and TV stations, high voltage lines etc. This affects our aura both as individuals and as society. We are now starting to learn about the deleterious effects of mobile phones – high frequency field effects adjacent to the brain. In addition, recent research from Sweden has shown that exposure to electromagnetic fields from Visual Display Units reduces blood levels of melatonin, a brain chemical that enhances mood and sleep. Low levels of melatonin are linked to lowered immune function.

The human energy field can be defined as an emanation from a person, not normally visible to the naked eye, that particularly encircles the head. Why is this? As we shall see, this is because the higher centres 'live' up in the head and throat areas. This part of the field is described as a cloud of light encircling the person or – in mystical terms – an envelope whose wholeness is controlled by the balance between the mind, body and spirit. Another reason is that clothing blocks the aura, making it more difficult to see.

The aura itself consists of subtle and more gross elements. It is often known commonly as the light seen around the heads of saints as portrayed so lovingly in the stained glass of churches. This is the aura in its most subtle form. However it also has other elements – less subtle and more mechanical – consisting of electrical and magnetic fields which have in some cases been measured by instruments.

Conventional scientific opinion is that the human body is mainly a chemical machine of hugely complex form. Literally thousands of chemicals are produced. However, evidence has accumulated over the last 200 years and particularly since the 1930's that the body is not only chemical in nature, but also comprises significant magnetic, electrical and energetic components.

These ideas go back at least to the time of Mesmer in the 1800's. He reported that animate and inanimate objects could be charged with a fluid, and that in general, 'living matter has a property susceptible to being acted on by earthly and celestial magnetic forces'. Mesmer postulated that the entire universe is filled with a fluid less perceptible than gas in which all matter is immersed, and that the fluid carries vibrations in its substance.

He suggested that the vibrations of this fluid, permeating as it did the entire universe, caused all existing physical phenomena. Mesmer, who was a physician

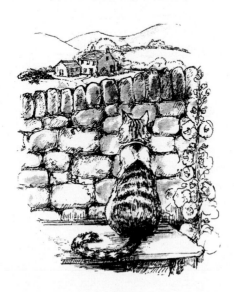

Many animals can sense the approach of their owner, or another animal even though they are too far away to be detected by the five senses. Do cats use their whiskers as antennae to detect electromagnetic fields?

and a natural scientist, also believed that each living body causes a direct influence upon other living bodies transmitted through a vibration of the ether.

Mesmer confirmed an earlier discovery that magnets had healing power, and it was in the course of such studies that he found that his hands emitted an energy which he termed 'animal magnetism', so named because it was found that its therapeutic effects were similar to that of physical magnetism of permanent magnets that Mesmer had previously worked with.

However, pioneers suffer from martyrdom. The opposition to Mesmer's ideas in official circles was so strong that for decades and centuries any physician or scientist who tried to introduce similar ideas into the community – even ideas that merely tried to show that there was an electromagnetic energy associated with the body – confronted condemnation.

The 'aura' is a very comprehensive and, some would say, nebulous topic. It is not the predominant colour that need concern us but the internal mechanisms. For example we speak of a 'highly charged' atmosphere. In the case of some human cases this is the literal truth. One man, Brian Williams of Cardiff, obtained notoriety. He was so full of electricity that he could light a lamp simply by rubbing it with his hand. Others are plagued with electric shocks and have to discharge before they touch others. A researcher, Vincent Gaddis, mentions the case of a 16-year old student in Maryland, USA, in 1890. When the tips of his fingers were dry, he could pick up heavy objects simply by touching them and pins would dangle from his open hand as though from a magnet.

In many respects electricity behaves like a fluid. Mesmer described it as OD or electric fluid. A current is a stream of electrons that carry a negative electric charge. When electricity accumulates on the human body as a result of friction as when we walk on a carpet, it may be at a potential of thousands of volts, though with a tiny charge.

Usually we are not aware of the electrical qualities inherent in nature and our bodies in particular because negative and positive charges exist in equal quantities around us, and their effects cancel out. Only when the two are separated – as when we touch a live mains wire – do we notice their effects.

It is not unreasonable to conclude that these interplays of voltages cause a concomitant field effect around the body. A magnet has a field. The blood, which circulates, contains an iron-bearing – magnetic – substance which has its own field properties.

Also during the 1800's, the famous German chemist and industrialist Baron von Reichenbach (1788–1869) made a substantial contribution by his discovery of paraffin and creosote. However, what consumed him more and more, occupying 30 years of this creative life, was his interest in the mysteries of electricity and magnetism. He became aware of a life-force associated with living people which he dubbed "odic force" or "od" for short, named after the Norse god Odin to suggest the idea of a force with a power that cannot be obstructed, quickly penetrates and courses through everything in the universe.

In order to make observations of the odic force, von Reichenbach used the services of many sensitives and clairvoyants. He found that the observed 'od' from magnets and human subjects exhibited many properties which were similar. He determined that the poles of a magnet not only exhibit the normal magnetic polarity but also a unique polarity associated with this "odic field". Magnets gave off a particularly bright light at the poles, the north being surrounded by a white light merging into layers of red, yellow, green and finally blue. The middle of the magnet gave off a glowing green haze, and the south pole an even brighter white than the north, merging into red. This energy was also observed to surround the human body, and in particular seen to flow from the finger tips. What is electricity? What is magnetism? We still do not know. The best definition was given by a distinguished scientist: "electricity is the way that nature behaves".

In addition to visual sightings, the clairvoyant subjects reported that such fields or auras felt "hot, and red or unpleasant" or "blue and cold and pleasant" to the touch.

Dr Wilhelm Reich became interested in a universal energy that he named 'orgone'. His studies as a psychiatrist and colleague of Freud took place in the early part of the 20th century. He studied the relationship of disturbances in the energy flow in the human body to various types of illness. He learned to identify and release energy blocks which cleared negative mental and emotional states.

In the period of the 1930's through to the 1950's he experimented with these energies using the latest electronic and medical instrumentation. He observed this energy pulsating in the sky and around all organic and indeed inanimate objects. He devised a variety of physical apparatuses for the study of this field, and learned to focus and concentrate this orgone energy which was used to charge objects.

In 1924 the French scientist Louis de Broglie made a discovery which earned him the Nobel Prize for 1929. He advanced the theory of wave properties of matter. According to his theory, around any object there exists an imperceptible, but real wave field. In multicavital structures, where the surface area of a solid body is large and, at the same time, intricately curved, these waves form and generate 'standing' waves with much smaller particles but with an increase in total energy. Thus, strengthening themselves by way of mutual overlapping in the cells (like an overtone in musical instruments), they form clusters – maximums of standing waves. This theory would explain some of the experiments described below.

In the 1930's, embryologist Dr. Harold Saxton Burr of Yale University, and his colleague Dr. F. Northrup devoted themselves to the examination of electromagnetic fields around living objects, and in 1935 published their work under the title *The Electro-Dynamic Theory of Life*. We can certainly consider this as a legitimate part of the aura, though it cannot be seen. They used an ultra-sensitive vacuum tube voltmeter which could measure voltages as small as one millionth of a volt between two points within or on a living system. They detected steady electric potential gradients on the surface of many different types of organisms which were

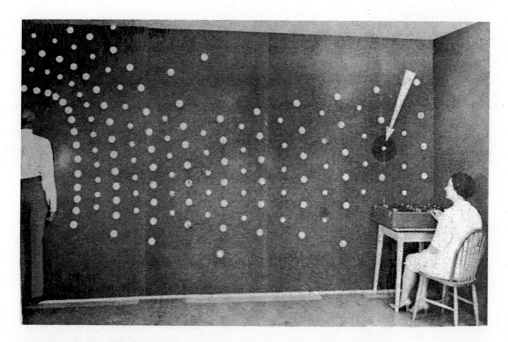

Early experiments of standing waves emanating from a human subject. These nodal points, as George De La Warr called them, are being detected by a portable multi-oscilloscope.

characteristic for each different species. In experiments with trees, they found that trees had bioelectric fields that varied in response not only to physiological activity, light intensities and moisture but also to changes in atmospheric electricity and geomagnetic field strength related to thunderstorms, sunspot cycles and moon phases.

In another set of experiments with human female subjects Dr. Burr measured the voltage differences between the cervix and a distant part of the body – usually the ankle. He found that there was an increased voltage difference lasting about 24 hours, which occured in the middle of the menstrual cycle.

Numerous names have been given to these electrical fields. Electromagnetic fields, electrostatic fields, electrodynamic fields. These are not different types of fields. The nomenclature arises from the different types of instruments used to measure the fields. A machine dependent on static forces would define the fields as electrostatic etc. Burr called these energy fields of living organisms L-fields (life fields or organizing fields). These fields give instructions to us as to how the body should grow – and stop growing! They exist independent of physical matter. They are subtle and three dimensional. They have magnitude and directional elements. They extend from the physical confines of the object and therefore cannot be measured in their entirety.

Apart from these natural life fields, Burr found another group of fields which were affected by a person's thoughts. These, Burr christened T-fields. These can be detected by the average person as an 'atmosphere' in a room, for example. Our

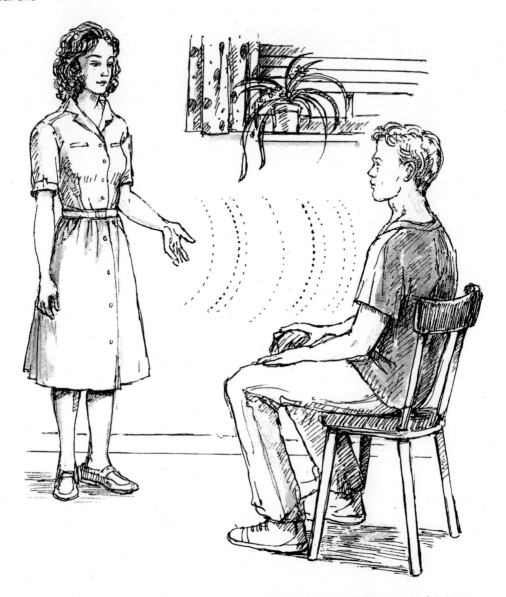

Using the aura instead of a machine to detect standing waves. See later in the book for details but anyone can do it. Focus on the person in front of you and move your left hand backwards and forwards until prickles are felt. Note how far away you are when the impressions are felt. IDEA – get a friend to do the same and see if they get the impressions in the same place.

nervous system is capable of detecting minute changes in voltage and is thus capable of resonating with other living systems in the vicinity. He also discovered that mentally unstable people displayed varied and erratic patterns in the voltage potential of their L-fields, and that it was possible to predict accurately the forthcoming reactions of seriously disturbed mental patients.

The nervous system of the human being is ideally suited to detecting such fields. This information is absorbed and programmed into the mind of the recipient, analysed, compared with what has gone before and identified as signal or noise.

On a wider level, Burr feels that since the field of living patterns are ordered, it must be part of an overall general pattern which represents the universe. It can be argued that the universe is itself an electrical field and that everything that exists in it is a subsidiary or component part of the total field. The idea is not new – religions have known this for millenia – Jesus, for example, said that we are all members one of another. But recent decades have seen the component fields – living forms – subject to scientific investigation and measurement. These living systems are not some extraneous creation imported into this universe but an integral part of the pattern. In short 'all the body is in the mind, but not all the mind is in the body'.

Research into the light emission properties of the body continues. In New York in 1969, a group of physicists, physicians, electronic and biological specialists amalgamated their efforts forming the Energy Research Group (including Drs. Richard Dobrin, Barbara Conway and John Pierrakos) with the aim of discovering if the human energy field has a physical reality.

This group, using state of the art instruments, observed the human body and attempted to determine the relationship between the observed radiation and physical and emotional illness and health.

They positioned two photomultiplier tubes in a light-tight room. This apparatus detects and amplifies low levels of light. The models were designed to respond to light in the visible and ultraviolet, but not in the infra-red part of the spectrum, and would therefore exclude variations of the natural heat from the body. The subjects stood 12 inches from the tubes which were aimed at the abdomen.

With the subjects, an average light emission of 15% above the background noise was recorded. This low light level – in the range of 20–200 photons per second – is within the range of human night vision. 90% of individuals gave a recordable signal at some level. Some subjects could increase the light emission by 100% simply by conscious effort. The subjects claimed to be projecting energy from either their solar plexus, their heads or their hands. Temperature in the darkroom was observed to be constant.

Another feature found with strong subjects was that the photomultiplier signal did not completely disappear when the subject left the darkroom. The signal decayed over a period of 15–20 minutes. This 'lag effect' has been observed by other investigators and has led to the conclusion that some form of energy has been left in the room by the subject.

Meditation increased the intensity of the subject's signal whilst intense thinking reduced the field intensity. In another experiment, a pregnant woman was seated on the floor of the darkroom with her body out of range of visibility of the photomultiplier tubes. A large signal was nonetheless recorded as if she were projecting or emitting a visible signal from her head and body. This effect supports the evidence for an emitted field. In other experiments, subjects were able to project their energy into the darkroom with visible increases in the observed signal.

The opposite type of effect was seen with others who decreased the observed

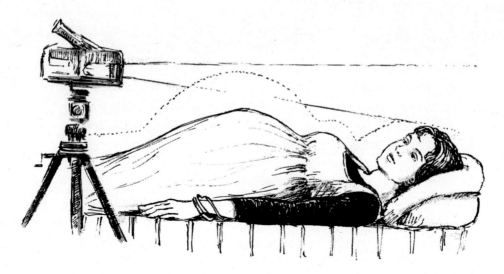

Experiments by the Energy Research Group, New York, detected an area of light over the womb of a pregnant female.

signal below the background level when they entered the room. This included one agitated subject who appeared to draw energy from her surroundings. The subjective impression of the experimenters was that she was "sucking energy" from the people whom she came into contact with.

Attempts to video the signal resulted in the sight of a thin pulsating field around the body. Several horn-shaped structures were seen in areas corresponding to what eastern literature describes as the chakras, or openings into which energy is reputed to flow into the body from the sea of energy that surrounds it.

Alexander Avshulumov, writing in a now defunct Russian bioenergetic journal in 1993, echos the views of many others when he comments on the use of the tremendous and diverse information given out by the human being, and its use in early diagnosis of problems. Living cells emit a very weak light in the ultraviolet part of the spectrum.

One of the most mysterious aspects of life was discovered in regeneration studies with salamanders early this century: the over-all pattern of the body is as much a part of the body as any individual cell or organ.

If you amputate the foreleg of a salamander, first the blastema (the undifferentiated cells) will develop. Then the blastema transforms itself into a new, complete foreleg. If you transplant the blastema early in its development, still undifferentiated, to the area of the hind leg, it will develop as a hind leg. If you wait a few weeks, while it is still an undifferentiated blastema, then transplant it, it will then develop into a foreleg.

Thus, the early blastema knows where it is, and the late blastema knows where it was.

Each part of the body, then, knows where it is in relation to the whole body. Under the Clockwork Paradigm, this is as impossible as the two photons in the EPR experiment being aware of each other. Now, we can rationally explain this mystery. This mystery of the body parts knowing where they are in relation to each other and to the whole has been known and described since early in this century. Only since the work of Dr. Becker can we feel confident about the answer.

Currently we know that there is an electromagnetic field in and around the body. We know that electromagnetic fields are excellent for storing, carrying, and processing information. It seems obvious that the over-all electromagnetic field itself carries this information of the body's shape and pattern. This information is probably stored as gradients within the field.

These electromagnetic gradients would activate the DNA in tissues such as blastemas to "tell" them what they need to know. In the case of salamander regeneration, it activates the genes which say "foreleg" or "hind leg" about halfway through the life of the blastema. This same process is almost certainly what is responsible for the development of the foetus as well as normal maintenance and healing of tissues.

One very important aspect of the body electric which has been taken for granted is the polarized cell membrane. Not only neurons, but every cell in the body has an electrical polarization across the membrane.

This electrical polarization across the cell membrane seems to be very small, so that the electrical aspect of it has been thought to be meaningless.

In fact, the actual electrical potential is 50 millivolts across a thickness of 50 Angstroms. This is a small amount of electricity over a very, very, very, very small distance. Angstroms are the measure for the size of atoms! The cell membrane's electrical potential corresponds to a voltage of one hundred thousand volts per centimetre, which is high voltage.

Good commercial insulators, such as porcelain, break down under a stress of seventy thousand volts per centimetre. This means that the electricity which holds our cells together is far from insignificant. The body is a high voltage mechanism.

So far, I have been emphasizing that the body has electrical characteristics in the way that we normally understand electricity – there are, for example, electromagnetic frequencies from the semi-conducting direct currents, and voltages across the cell membrane.

Now, remember that each molecule, each atom, is itself a true electromagnetic process in its own right. Atoms are not solid particles. DNA is not a just chain of particles, but a chain of swirling electromagnetic energies. The same is true for proteins, carbohydrates, fats, and water. Each of these electromagnetic entities has its own frequencies, its own rhythms of pulsation. Each of these electromagnetic entities carries a lot of information in their electromagnetic fields.

Each of these electromagnetic entities contributes to the whole of your being. Each is a part of your life energy in a very literal way. We are pure energy.

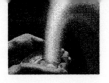

CHAPTER TWO

THE AURA AND ITS STRUCTURE

The aura is reputed to consist of various layers. And some analysis of layers can be helpful provided it is not carried to extremes. Immediately outside the physical body there is the 'etheric double' which is a replica of the physical body that it envelopes, thus becoming an intermediate layer between the body and the inner aura. This is where indications of physical health appear. Next to the etheric double is the inner aura which reacts very sensitively to the slightest emotional changes. When you feel sad or happy, or when you are laughing, changes take place in the form of specific rhythms of vibrations, the density of the field or hues of its colour.

The outer aura is more responsive to changes such as pregnancy and certain emotional states, according to the aura researcher Oscar Bagnall. Readers are referred to the excellent classics on the subject by Annie Besant and C.W. Leadbeater including *Thought forms* and *Man Visible and Invisible*.

The shape of the aura changes with mental and physical health. Two Russian scientists – the engineer and inventor Yuri Kravchenko and the physician Nikolai Kalashenko – have developed an original instrument christened the phase aurometer. This is a highly sensitive instrument for the remote measurement of the electromagnetic radiation of any object, biological included. Different pathologies were characterized by a differing electromagnetic field intensity. The shape of the radiations indicate the person's health status. Chakras are measured from both the front and the back. Recorded signals appear to be in the thermal microwave and Extra High Frequency range (1–10 GHz), and the infrared and optical range but none in the 10–100,000 KHz range. Hence the human body is broadcasting on certain frequencies very much like a transmitting aerial. This forms the basis for instant so-called telepathic conversation and communication. Due to the pollution of our environment this inherent ability is much more difficult to use, though by no means impossible. Belief in the aura is no longer in the realm of superstition. It is entering the realm of science as the amount and quality of evidence increases.

THE AURA AND ITS FUNCTIONS

The aura is the vital interface between our physical body and the human environment. We have all experienced that during a personal depression restaurant waiters ignore us. This is because our aura has withdrawn. All of us sense the aura whether we care to admit it or not. The term 'good vibes' which has come into common usage is indicative of this growing awareness of sensitivity. We know immediately when we are uncomfortable in a certain place or in the company of certain people. Thoughts imprint themselves into the physical surroundings, giving an atmosphere which few can avoid picking up.

Modern technological thinkers give no credence to the idea of an aura. It is an optional extra to the essential business of earning a living. Nevertheless, if we are to behave intelligently, we need to take all factors of our existence into consideration. Apart from the constancy of mystic and religious teaching, science shows us that this other type of matter needs to be taken into consideration. The aura is the link between us, our body, mind, soul and spirit and the universe of energy. There are many functions of the aura, but two of the main ones are protection, and the means of giving information about our physical mental and psychological condition. Because every living thing has an aura, this information is 'broadcast' on a 24-hour basis. We have also learned that any radiation carries with it all the information about its source. Our will has nothing to do with this. It reveals the extent of our integration.

PARTS OF THE AURA – THE VARIOUS BODIES

To refer to each aspect of our existence in terms of 'bodies' may be confusing. Only the physical body has a clearly defined form and density. All other bodies – the subtle bodies – have forms but no substance. You can put your hand through it. The cosmic body or corpus, expressed as individual, group and cultural consciousness – it has no location or form. It is everywhere at once. There is no feeling of 'self' or 'other'.

A human aura can be viewed as a 'body'. It holds no views or prejudices. It reports what is going on within the human consciousness on the physical, mental, emotional and spiritual level. It is a composite which can be broken down into elements for analysis and surveyance. Imagine film transparencies taken by cameras with different filters of the same subject. If all the transparencies are superimposed, then the total will have different degrees of density and consistency. Energy bodies cannot be seen meaningfully in isolation. Let us have a look at the various aspects of the aura according to function and subtlety.

The physical body

The first of our bodies is the physical body. This, in esoteric terms, is the lowest aspect of our life, the grossest means of expression for our soul. In material terms it is the vehicle that enables our survival on this planet. In its divisions we see a reflection of the inner levels of consciousness. We shall discuss how the physical body relates to the chakras later on, but meanwhile, we shall view the physical body as the 'body temple' divided into parts.

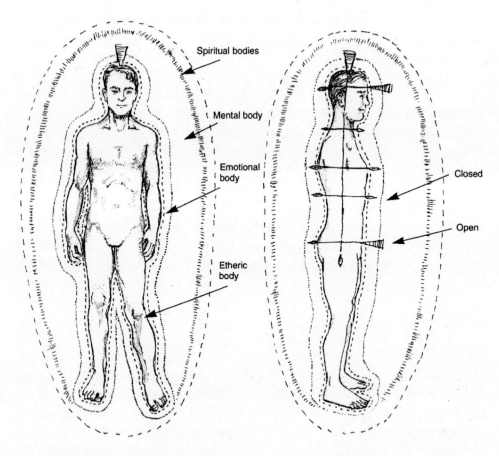

Spiritual bodies

Mental body

Emotional body

Etheric body

Closed

Open

'LAYERS OF THE AURA'.

The outer court of the temple contains the organs of assimilation and procreation. The diaphragm represents a veil between the higher and lower levels of consciousness. The chest cavity symbolizes the inner court of the temple containing the organs of the heart and lungs whose function is to bring the life-force into circulation. Through the bridge of the neck lies the holy of holies, the dwelling place of the spirit. This contains the organs of spiritual perception, the pituitary and pineal glands. Every physical organ is a metaphor or symbol for deep and complex spiritual truths.

The etheric body

The etheric body lies between the subtle mental bodies and the physical body and its world. It is a mediating, vitalizing body. The etheric body is the framework on which the physical framework is built. The etheric body has three basic functions which are all closely related. It acts as a receiver, assimilator and transmitter of prana. Prana is the universal life force that vitalizes all forms in all kingdoms of nature. These energies streaming in from the sun are absorbed by the etheric body though a series of small force centres and then passed on to the spleen, where the vital essence of the sun is modified and then circulated to vitalize the physical body. The etheric body of man can be considered receptive or negative in respect to solar radiations, and as positive or expansive in respect to the physical body.

The etheric body is thus the field where spiritual and physical worlds meet. It gives rise to the 'health' aura, that narrow band of energy surrounding the body. The interplay of energies build and sustain our glands and the nervous system, distributing prana and energizing the physical form.

This body is sometimes referred to as the 'etheric double', because its shape is similar to that of the physical form. It underlies and interpenetrates every atom, molecule and cell of the physical body. The five physical senses work through the etheric body enabling us to function in time and space.

To the clairvoyant it is seen as a fine network of energy streams. Those familiar with the work of Carlos Castaneda know that it is described as "fibres of light looking like white cobwebs, luminous and bristling out in all directions, putting man in touch with all things". These numerous fibres of energy – which the Indians call nadis, form the archetypal pattern or framework upon which the physical body is built.

The emotional body

This subtle body is the stage on which the interplay of emotional energies takes place. It is sometimes called the astral body due to its sparkling appearance provided it is not clouded by negative emotions. In this, our own personal heaven and hell, we experience the pull of opposite emotions.

The symbol of the emotional body is water. As you cannot see the bottom of a lake when the water is choppy, so you cannot obtain tranquillity unless the emotional body is calm. This body is particularly visible to the clairvoyant in the form of interweaving colours. It is from this body that out of body experiences (OBE's) take place. These can happen during moments of great stress, during anaesthetic or at the point of death.

The mental body

There are a number of divisions to this mind or mental body. There is the lower mind – the reasoning principle that applies logic and common sense. It is a reservoir of learned and acquired knowledge and the ability to discriminate. It can have an adverse effect on the astral body if too active.

Negative and habitual thought patterns pollute the astral body. It can lead to separatist and divisive thinking and has been described as 'the slayer of the real'. Mentally, people can block light and truth most effectively! Negative thoughts such as hatred, prejudice, selfishness and greed cause forms that accumulate in the lower part of the aura in coarse and dull colours. According to clairvoyants, people who are preoccupied with sluggish thoughts create an ovoid field like a pear shape with a large part on the bottom. Clear thoughts produce this shape in reverse.

Another aspect of the mental body is the higher abstract mind which conveys spiritual truths and reflects divine love. Here resides pure reason and the intuitive faculties. Higher thoughts on the other hand move to the upper part of the aura and are seen as clear, bright radiant colours. We speak of 'sharp as a pin' or 'dull as ditch water' when describing others. These communicate even to those who are not aware of any psychic gift.

WHAT IS AN 'INTEGRATED' PERSON?

At this stage, let's see how our knowledge links up with the notion of personal integrity. Does integration have any connection with the aura? To 'integrate' means the completion of a thing imperfect and incomplete in itself by the addition of parts and the combination of these parts into a whole. It's from the Latin *integrare* – to make whole. Our left brain is connected with logical thinking, reason, the protection of our territory, calculation, the intellect in general. Our right brain has more abstract functions such as intuition, feeling and emotions. Our Western hemisphere is left-brain dominated. We make a god of possessions, acquisition and materialism. These crush our intuitive, transcendent and wholistic functioning. In addition our brain can be divided into three types of functioning. The 'reptile brain', the oldest primitive part concerning territory, aggression, self-defence; the limbic part which is concerned with emotions, feelings and the newest part – the neo-cortex, which is related to the higher functions such as altruism. This triune brain straddles both the left and right hemisphere. The neo-cortex is linked with the higher chakras, the limbic centred round the heart and the instinctive territorial reptile brain is centred round and linked with the base chakra.

WHAT HAPPENS IF THE AURA IS INTEGRATED?

We can see that with the complexity of our consciousness, keeping the whole thing stable is not something that happens automatically. We can develop counter-productive habits without realizing it. As the English writer Samuel Johnson said 'The chains of habit are too weak to be felt until they are too strong to be broken'. An integrated aura is the fullest expression of the individual and provides a 'layer' or 'glove' of light around us. What practical implications does this have? Our 'wholeness' or 'integrity' manifests in a whole aura. If you can imagine a glove of light with no gaps or tears – that is the aura at its best. The benefit is that others' disharmony – or lack of integrity – cannot reach you when you are in this condition. Gross thoughts cannot penetrate the material of the aura. If you recall the first time you fell in love, everything was wonderful, glowing, positive. Your feet hardly touched the ground. In this case under the powerful influence of love, the aura was – if only temporarily – whole.

Another person could have a dispute or argument in the same room and you would not be affected. If, however, you yourself were in a bad condition you would suffer and be negatively affected by the presence of the other party and their discord. This would be because your own aura would have holes or gaps in it and other vibrations could find an easy admittance. That is why happiness and joy is so important.

The other equally important function of the aura is to give information about us.

The existence of telepathy – namely the transmission of thoughts from one person to another – has been established conclusively by many researchers including Dr. J. B. Rhine of Duke University. The distance between the sender and receiver makes no difference. You can conduct an experiment between two people one thousand miles apart and it can be just as successful as one conducted in adjacent rooms of the same building. It is a matter of conjecture how this works.

Prof. Vasiliev, Professor of Physiology in the University of Leningrad, demonstrated the same, that thought acts at a distance and penetrates all obstacles. Neither concrete walls, lead chambers or Faraday cages made the slightest difference. He established in a series of double blind experiments that there was an energetic connecting link between two people situated a considerable distance apart. He showed that a thought in one mind produced an effect across space in another mind. This shows that thought behaves like a field.

In physics, the equivalent is the effect at a distance of a magnet on iron filings. Fields resonate at a distance. To this fact we owe broadcast telecommunications, where one circuit is set to resonate with another circuit. Modifications in one are reflected in modifications in the other and thus information is sent. However, the fields referred to above are the same which Harold Saxton Burr later called T-fields (thought fields). They also appear to have the property of attaching themselves to any kind of matter of any shape or size. This is commonly evidenced by the blessing or cursing of objects, and by the effect on the atmosphere of a building where a terrible tragedy has taken place. The size of the object is immaterial – it can either be a wedding ring, or a six story building. These curious and unique timeless fields are independent of matter and can travel through space without attenuation.

Not only people but places and even objects can have an aura for good or for bad. I recall a story of a friend of mine who bought a second-hand ring from a shop. After some time, he noticed a small lump. He went to the doctor who diagnosed the early stage of cancer. He by chance went to a sensitive. She took one look at him and said "why are you wearing that ring?" He returned to the shop with the ring. On telling his story the jeweller laughed. "You are the third person to bring the ring back", he said. "No one can wear it. It was from the estate of an old lady who died from cancer!" True or apocryphal, the vibrations coming from an object are used in the ancient skill of psychometry. If objects remember things they have been in contact with, how much more will the human aura 'remember'?

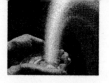

CHAPTER THREE

PERCEIVING THE AURA

We all have skills and abilities which can be developed if we choose. Many abilities possessed by so-called primitive people, for example the aborigines, have been lost in more advanced technical society. The aura, or at least a part of it, can be photographed by machines (as in Kirlian Photography) or evidentially (as with the 'aura camera'), or with light enhancing devices such as a photo multiplier tube, or with the human eye, aided or unaided.

In recent scientific history, the phenomena of light – or bioluminescence – has been discovered more by chance, a by-product of other work. A pioneer in subtle energies was William Roentgen, a medical researcher at St. Thomas' Hospital in London. He pioneered scientific research on 'rays of an unknown origin' which he called 'X-rays'. He found them to have among the shortest frequencies in the electromagnetic spectrum. As we all know, the X-ray has become an accepted diagnostic method in medicine. The X-ray has the energy to go through muscular tissue, seeing obstacles in its path, and exposing photosensitive film.

A colleague of Roentgen, Walter Kilner, a medical electrician and member of London's Royal College of Surgeons, was convinced of the reality of the human aura. In his book *The Human Aura* – based on four years' work – he wrote "there cannot be the least doubt of the reality of the existence of an aura enveloping a human being, and this will be in a short time a universally accepted fact".

He speculated that 'magnetic radiations', as he thought they were, might be more detectable by sensitives as the radiation seemed to belong to the ultra violet frequency which is at the extreme end of the visible spectrum. Visible light comprises only a tiny part of the whole electromagnetic wave spectrum which runs from the very long 10 to the power of 9 for direct current electricity to the extremely short 10 to the power of – 14 for gamma rays. The wavelength of light is between 360 nanometres and 780 nanometres.

He developed so-called aura goggles which consisted of glasses which enclose the eyes with thick layered lenses consisting of dicyanin dye. He trained experimenters to stare at the subject against a grey background. According to Kilner (who may have been clairvoyant himself) he could actually see a cloud of radiation extending out about six to eight inches and showing distinct colours. Fatigue, diseases or mood could alter the size and colour; this radiation was also affected by magnetism, hypnosis and electricity. Kilner found that some subjects could change their colours at will.

HOW DO WE SENSE SUBTLE ENERGIES?

Let's start from where people are. Everyone has one sense that they tend to prefer using. Sight, hearing, and touch are the most common. When you receive information psychically, it will tend to appear in the form that is easiest for you to understand. Most of the information will appear to you through your strongest sense, the one you are comfortable with. If you are a visual person, you will mostly receive images. If you learn more easily through hearing, you will hear voices or words telling you the information. If you learn more through touch, you will gain information by feeling yourself in the situation you want information about and even by using your nervous system. You may be an intuitive person, who simply knows the information without it taking any specific form. Or you may feel emotionally that something in particular is right. Regardless of your strengths and preference, you will probably receive some information in every form, so be open to all of it. However, information is transferred best when all psychic senses are open to receive as much as possible.

Some see the aura naturally. The great seer Edgar Cayce writing his book on auras wrote "Ever since I can remember, I have seen colours in connection with people. I do not remember a time when the human beings I encountered did not register on my retina with blues and greens and reds gently pouring from their heads and shoulders. It was a long time before I realized that other people did not see these colours. It was a long time before I heard the word 'aura' and learned to apply it to this phenomenon. To me it was commonplace. I do not even think of people except in connection with their auras. I see them change in my friends and loved ones as time goes by. Sickness, dejection, love and fulfilment. These are all reflected in the aura and for me the aura is the weather vane of the soul. It shows me the way that the winds of destiny are blowing."

Children sometimes see colours around people as a fluid, multihued field which Cayce related to people's moods. Seeing colours or the ability to be telepathic is a natural gift which seems to disappear in children after about the age of six. It is most important that parents encourage their children to share dreams and experiences, and not to laugh or deride them. This should give us a clue as to the state of mind in which we can see the aura. The innocence and unself-consciousness of a child is vital. It cannot be forced. Who knows, you may not be ready to see auras yet. If in doubt, leave it! If you had the ability to see all the good and the bad round your fellow human beings it would indeed be a burden.

Prehistoric man relied on this uncomplicated sensitivity and depended heavily on his ability to see or sense the aura. To him it meant survival, the one dominant theme that pervaded his life. It was essential for him to know what was going on

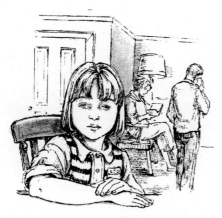

Children often lose their natural psychic ability at the age of six.

not only in his immediate environment but at a distance, through a form of radiatory energy affinity which he could use to determine the presence of game at a distance or identifying the location of predators. He lived in an unpolluted environment in which all life forms – man, animal and vegetation constantly interacted in terms of reciprocal energy exchanges.

Man has a unique ability – that is to add the process of thought to energy field identification at a distance. He moved into a position of dominance and learned to probe into and decipher these auric fields to his own advantage. Animals do the same to an extent but are limited in their intelligence.

First it would appear necessary to have some light in order to perceive the aura unaided. An aura cannot be seen in a completely blacked out room. The detection apparatus of the human body is much more subtle than we realize and multi-faceted. It may well be that our naked eye is more geared to detecting ultraviolet light than we realize. Detection mechanisms in our eyes comprise rods (around 18 million of them) and cones (about 3 million). They are geared to pick up different wavelengths of light. Cones see visible light. Rods do not recognize colours – everything looks greyish blue. The rods are not affected by red light or light with longer wavelengths, but are stimulated by ultraviolet light.

In addition there is the pineal gland, expressed through the third eye, which may have a contributing influence. This gland, according to many philosophers, is the 'seat of the soul', acting as a link between the visible and invisible worlds. It enables us to understand life with a clear perspective and maintain hope, faith and balance in a confusing and changing world. It allows us to perceive the inner qualities of others. Descartes believed that "In man, soul and body touch each other only at a single point, the pineal gland in the head". Prayer and meditation is said to bring about an awakening of intuitive perception. This gland has been likened to an alchemical retort, which releases its spiritual essence into man when the dross has been burnt out from his personality. He is slowly but surely transformed into a bearer of light. It is not possible to open the third eye in the way that we open our normal eyes. The shock would be too great and damage would occur to the whole aura.

WHAT AM I SEEING WITH?

There is more than one way of 'seeing'. The first is to use the full capacity of the naked eye. The unaided eye sees what we know as the colours of the spectrum.

In exceptional circumstances this may be extended to the infrared and ultraviolet ends of the spectrum. The second is to use the third eye, or pineal gland which some say is the seat of the soul. It would be most unusual to view all the colours described in this book. They are more likely to be felt. However, very occasionally, a developed person may see this surround in full colour. This changes according to health and mood. The third method – much beloved by detractors of parapsychological phenomenon, is inner projection. Typically in a state of relaxation the inner eye perceives an object which appears to have objective reality when in fact it is only happening within the cranium. The fourth type of seeing is that class of phenomenon due to distortions in the physical environment. An example is a person in the desert seeing a mirage, which is light waves from an event elsewhere transposing themselves on to a physical horizon much distant from the original event. We are concerned primarily with third eye sight and that phenomenon occuring just outside the visible part of the spectrum, or of such a low intensity that normal photographic apparatus cannot detect it.

METHODS TO DEVELOP AURIC SIGHT

The most important rule – be positive! Just because you have never seen an aura does not mean that you are unable to see one. The very impulse to try may mean that you are ready for it. This phenomenon can appear to some people all of a sudden; for others it is a gradual process. Do not force the pace. When you try too hard you will automatically switch to focused vision. The muscles of the eye will then fatigue and you will see a 'false aura' which is a flat colour, not translucent like the real aura. It will be the opposite or complement of the colour of the clothes of the subject – for instance, a person wearing a red shirt will create a false green aura, a purple shirt will create a false yellow aura.

The majority of people who talk about seeing the aura report that a sighting took place when least expected. It might have been a shape round a dying patient, or the sight of a 'double' when someone was in a dangerous or dramatic situation. No advance warning is given.

Try this simple experiment. When you feel in a relaxed mood, find a room with a wall colour that is not distracting. Grey, white, and dark colours such as brown are good. There should be no objects in the room in your field of view. Stand facing the wall without any bright sunlight and hold your hands in front of you – about 10 inches apart. You may see slight traces of smoke-like energy coming from the tips of your fingers. Try this for about a minute. You need to be patient because according to Walter Kilner, one of the pioneers of aura viewing, it is primarily the rods that do the viewing, and they work more slowly than cones. If nothing happens do not worry. Relax and try it again. Let things flow without forcing anything. You can also try it outside. Raise your arm and study it against the sky. Lie down, and look at your legs. Make sure the skin is bare when you do this.

How to see the aura of another person

The next exercise involves another person. Ask a friend to stand in front of you about 5 metres away. Again, make sure any light in the room is not too bright and that shafts of sunlight are not crossing your gaze. It is most important not to look directly at the subject. Look at them briefly, then look to the side and behind them. If you are worried that the friend will become bored, share this with them. There is no way you should feel foolish, or a failure, or both. Incidentally, experiments are more successful in the evening because the experimenter is tired, relaxed and a little dreamy. These are the ideal conditions.

There is an important question. Should the subject be clothed? Since colour, even white, reacts with the aura of the subject and will flood it with colour. Even neutral coloured clothes will dim the aura making it difficult to see. However in real life lack of clothing is not practical, so concentrate on the outline of the person. Do not look at them.

Music has a big effect on the aura. Ask a friend to wear a headset and play music that they like. This will energize the aura. Contrast this with playing music they cannot stand and observe the difference in their aura.

The importance of good record keeping

It cannot be over-emphasized how important it is to record what you see. It is so clear at the time that you think to yourself – how could I possibly forget it. But ... you do! As experiment follows experiment the detail of the earlier one fades, and that's the time when you kick yourself for not making a note of it. A quite ordinary day can turn into an extraordinary one without giving warning. For general recording purposes a notebook is good, a tape recorder is better. Leave it running whilst you work and recount as your experiences emerge.

There is another point about making records. The mind tends to dismiss phenomena it cannot understand. Yet the most important events are those that do not fit into any category, the contradictions, the anomalies. If you have thoughts or impressions or symbols – or even smells – make a note of them. They will, in all probability, fit into a pattern later. I remember once when I was engaged fulltime in some experiments with Kirlian Photography. I was photographing cauliflower. I cut one up into small pieces and placed the result in a

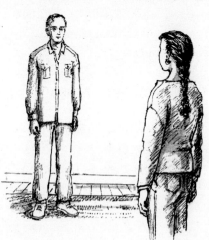

Attempting to see the aura of another person can best be done under conditions of relaxation.

plastic bag. I exposed the bag to a high voltage field on a sheet of photographic paper 4 inches × 5 inches. To my annoyance the whole paper was covered with yellow energy. Thinking that there was a photographic fault, I repeated the experiment twice more and with the same, though slightly less intense, result. Then, about five minutes later, made a third attempt. This time the photo had gone back to 'normal' with a few flares in the immediate vicinity of the bag. The interesting fact was that the photographic method was identical. I had made a mistake in attributing the 'superfluous' effect to a fault. It was showing me that a burst of energy accompanied the cutting up of the cauliflower.

HOW CAN I INCORPORATE AND DEVELOP THE THIRD EYE?

We cannot really separate the use of the third eye, from our perceptive mechanisms in general. Like any form of perception, there is only one way of developing the third eye and that is by practice. When you try the above experiment, feel yourself looking with your third eye also. This is an area of the forehead that tends to be psychically sensitive. To find it, close your eyes and feel your focus shift up slightly. Open and close your eyes a few times to find this shift. Don't roll your eyes backward to look up; this will just cause a headache! Once you are confident of where the focus shift is, try letting your focus shift up in the same way – but with your eyes open. Do it gently; don't force it. This should give the sensation of looking out of your eyes and out of your mind/forehead at the same time.

WHAT CAN I EXPECT TO SEE?

Don't worry about seeing in colour. Very often, shadowy shapes are seen in the first instance. The aura is like the layers of an onion but with each layer reaching from the very centre of a person outward. Observe the shape, texture and solidity of different auras to find out how you experience those things. Shape and texture tend to show the attitude of the person towards other people who are standing close to them; often a very sharp border and a solidly shaped aura show someone who is decisive about how close people can be to them, in other words, it is about personal space.

You may see your friend's aura reaching to a plant or a loved object. Do not be surprised at anything you see. There are no limits! You may see evidence of disease. This shows up in the aura in many different ways, sometimes days or weeks before any physical symptoms. An ear infection, for example, will show up as a shadow over the ear. As the infection takes hold, it will become infused with red and orange flecks.

HOW DO I KNOW IF I AM SEEING SOMETHING REAL?

Look past the object whose aura you want to see, using your eyes gently to see and keeping your focus lifted to the third eye area also. If you begin to see lines of colour around the object, you can check to see if they are an actual aura by looking away. If you see after-images that look like the lines you saw, it's not an aura. After-images are a biological effect of the eyes, from eye strain. To keep after-images from building up, blink fairly often and don't look at one thing for too long. As your aural vision improves you will not need to look at an object for very long to see an aura.

Don't be afraid of looking away when you think you can see an aura. If it is a real aura, it will be there when you look back and refocus on it. If it is not there then it is merely an after image. In this case it is useful to look away so you clear that image out of your eyes. Just close your eyes for a moment or two. When you stop seeing the image on the inside of your eyes, the image is cleared and you can go back to seeing the aura.

WHAT IF I DO NOT SEE ANYTHING?

Maybe you are trying too hard. Some people spend an hour trying to see something. The moment they give up they relax and the aura may appear right in front of your eyes. It is worth persisting, so why not have a break, go and do something enjoyable, and come back for another try. Like most things in life, practise makes perfect. You will find that each time you try, you see more.

Children are often better at seeing the aura. They are not self-conscious and take such things for granted. It is important never to laugh at a child who says they see things.

The aura is photosensitive and can expand to many times its normal size in sunlight. The aura in total can be likened to a tree. Energy and nutrition is drawn up through the root and fed through the trunk to the branches and leaves. The aura also absorbs energy from other sources around it such as sunlight, plants and other people. Therefore if you are trying to see the aura of another, get them to stand outside in bright sunlight first and then come in and stand in front of you.

Still no success. Don't worry. Such gifts are a mixed blessing. If we were to be able to see the aura surrounding everyone all the time, we would be in a mental hospital within a short time. Very few people in Western Society, even practising clairvoyants, are advanced and clear enough to view the whole aura. For the average person, sightings come in flashes. There are many very skilled and competent people who have never seen an aura, yet their contribution to society is substantial.

CAN THE AURA OF OTHER CREATURES BE DETECTED?

Viktor Grebennikov is a member of the Entomological Society of the Academy of Sciences specializing in the study of bees. He lives and works in Novosibirsk. He writes "In the spring of 1993, while searching for something on my instrument-cluttered laboratory table, I accidentally passed my hand over a container full of debris from the old nests of the subterranean sweat bee which I had gathered where bee colonies were concentrated. The beehive fragments resembled lumps of compressed clay with countless closet-cells placed side by side in an underground clustered structure. And so, while over these long-since lifeless fragments of hives, my hand suddenly felt warmth and some kind of prickling or twitching in the fingers. I was loath to trust my own senses, and once more passed my palm over the cells – again I felt warmth and tremors of a sort in my fingertips and joints. By moistening and earthing the fragments, I ascertained that the cause of these phenomena was not electricity. An extremely accurate thermometer confirmed that temperature was not the cause either. An apparatus highly sensitive to ultrasonic frequencies detected nothing." Grebennikov asked colleagues to hold their hands over the fragments and received over 200 pieces of evidence. Many experienced warmth, burnings, a puff of warm wind, a prickling sensation and compression. Others maintained that the hand was pushed upwards and its weight lessened (or on the contrary drawn downwards – having been made heavier). There were cases of temporary muteness and cramps during which it was as if the fingers were being twisted. Some test-subjects experienced a sour taste in the mouth as though they has touched a battery to their tongue, a burning in the throat, and a metallic after-taste. One person felt giddiness, another's breath was "taken away" and a third experienced blocked ears. The subjects were a complete cross-section including labourers, school children, agronomists and science workers.

It was noted that the radiations passed through any barrier – cardboard, metal or a brick wall – freely and with ease, as if there were no obstacle there at all. This is impressive but not incredible. Full or partial penetrability is characteristic of many physical fields – magnetic, electric and gravitational.

The above is a painstaking and thorough investigation of what most people can feel with a little practise and mental focus. Let it be said that many more people can feel the aura than see it. I recall one of the first exercises that drew my attention to the reality of the aura in the world of nature. On a residential weekend at the suggestion of the leader, a group of us stood around a syca-more tree about six feet from it. We stood with our palms uppermost and sent warm thoughts of greeting to it. The tree was alive. I pointed my hands towards the centre, and noticed that my palms were hot – as if an electric fire was focused on them. On impulse I turned my hands through 90% and the effect diminished.

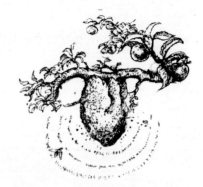

I continued to point my palms towards the tree. The prickles in my hand increased. I walked back and forth from the tree and I

BEES' NEST *Both bees' nests and bee substances exude a vibration which can be detected by non-trained members of the public.*

noticed that these impressions varied according to the distance from the tree. Some of the prickles were in the palm, others along the fingers and yet more on the back of the hand. I was to realize that my hand comprised a 'map' and could be programmed to receive information very much like a computer.

How to try this for yourself

Find an open area with trees far from pylons, houses and curious spectators! Dress in loose clothing. Make sure you have had no alcohol the same day. Spend some time in the area becoming attuned. Relax your mind and think of pleasant thoughts. It helps if you have someone with you that is on the same wavelength. They will not interfere with your experiment and will be available if you want to talk about it.

Using your intuition, hold your hands up, palms facing outwards, towards a tree that you feel some sympathy for. Take a few deep breaths and start about 20 metres from the tree. You may feel something straight away but allow a little longer if you do not. Try moving your hands slightly backwards and forwards. Whatever you notice – warmth or prickles or cold or shaking or electric lines, do not dismiss it. Everything is significant. This is the basis of an original method of diagnosis discussed later in this book.

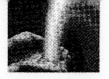

CHAPTER FOUR

THE AURA COLOURS AND THEIR MEANING

PROBLEMS OF VALIDATION

I do not recall reading of a case when a number of witnesses to a psychic phenomena reported seeing exactly the same thing. It is highly unlikely that even two people will observe the same colour or shape effect with an aura. We are all made in a unique way and all function differently. We see the auras of others through our own energy field, and in the real world it is likely to be distorted by our own predispositions. If I look at a landscape through a red filter, all colours will have their red element taken out of them. Sublimity, spiritual elevation and objectivity is required for accurate observation. That is why we as sensitives and those in the helping professions should seek to purify ourselves, our motives and emotions. It is for similar reasons that therapists and psychiatrists undergo a period of personal analysis before becoming qualified.

The association of light, particularly white light, with goodness and holiness is featured in all religious literature. Matthew, writing in the period after the death of Jesus Christ, reminds of his words "the lamp of the body is the eye. If your eyes are sound, you will have light for your whole body; if the eyes are bad, then the whole body will be in darkness. If then the only light you have is darkness, the darkness is doubly dark."

The use of the singular with the word 'eye' is significant. Could this refer to the third eye, or the pineal gland, which many psychics and sensitives think is the seat of the soul?

THE ENDOCRINE SYSTEM

Research into the pineal gland (Roney-Dougal, 1989) shows that the pineal gland is physiologically linked with the endocrine glands in the body, and that these endocrine glands are to be found at precisely the points which the yogis call the chakra points. This is very significant especially as the physiological functions of these endocrine glands correspond closely with the functions that the yogis ascribe to the chakras.

The pineal gland is considered to be the third eye, the psychic centre and I have found that the pineal gland produces a neurochemical which is hallucinagenic and is chemically similar to the active principle found in a vine used by Amazonian Indians to induce a psi-conductive state of consciousness. They use the vine specifically for psychic purposes. The pineal gland is considered by the yogis to be the command chakra linked to all the other chakras, and this is also true of the pineal gland in its chemical role in that it regulates the functions of all the other endocrine glands through its hormone melatonin.

As the mental, physical and spiritual state of a person is evolving all the time, so the colours do not remain constant. It is interesting to see how common phrases have entered into our language especially where negative emotions are concerned. We speak of being green with envy, black with depression and red with anger – even a 'fit of the blues!' We all have a subliminal awareness of the importance of colour in the aura.

From seeing the colours of the human aura, clairvoyants can tell about the emotional and spiritual state of the subject, including disease and imbalance. The use of the word clairvoyant, originally a pragmatic word, was derived from the French 'seeing clearly', a combination of two words 'clair' + 'voyant'. In this modern reductionist world the word is sometimes used in a judgmental way, describing a person who makes somewhat suspect claims to a gullible audience, engaging in wish fulfilment.

WHAT DO THE COLOURS MEAN?

There is no standard scale of colours verifiable by science, but general agreement exists amongst clairvoyants concerning the meanings of colours, which are by no means limited to the pure colours of the spectrum.

Annie Besant and C. W. Leadbeater in their book *Thought Forms* describe not only the predominant colour in the aura to which they ascribe meaning, but a variety of shapes associated with 'sudden fright', 'greed for drink', 'at a street accident' etc. These take geometric forms. Bessant and Leadbeater say that the body under the impulse of thought throws off a vibrating portion of itself, shaped by the nature of the vibrations, and this gathers from the surrounding atmosphere matter similar to itself in fineness from the elemental essence of the mental world. We have a combination of two factors – the overall colour of the aura, and the effect of thought currently going on.

Although the whole is very complex, the following will suffice for the beginner.

These are the colours associated with predominant states:

White. This is very rare and associated with a very highly spiritually evolved being. From the point of view of physics, white light is split up into all colours of the spectrum by a prism. White can be seen, symbolically, as all human qualities in balance and harmony. In the Bible, saints and holy people were 'arrayed in white raiment'. White is symbolic of purity, spirituality, God centredness. A person with a white aura heals naturally by their very presence. They are automatically protected from the force of evil. However, such people are often shy, lacking in the methodology of the ways of the world, finding living in big cities a particular stress.

Violet. Intuition and psychic ability, spiritual activity or information, trance mediumship, transmutation, therapeutic healing, protection, heart or stomach trouble, arrogance, superiority.

Indigo is the midway stage between dark blue and violet. It is the intuitive and spiritual in combination. It is a good stimulator for the third eye. If you mix dark blue with bright red you obtain violet. It concerns the psychic and spiritual faculty, regality and spiritual power arising from knowledge and occult pre-eminence. This represents activated knowledge which delimits the consciousness. On the physical level, violet assists with the healing of skin eruptions and the destruction of germs.

Blue is linked with creative and spiritual people and indicates clear channels to the spiritual realm. There are many hues of blue and a colour chart would be the ideal method of demonstrating them. For example dark navy blue indicates an inpouring of information from a deep pool of knowledge. It is linked with intuitive people and psychics display this blue. An interesting blue is that of the sky on a clear blue day. It is associated with the desire to learn, stimulation by something that is important for the evolution. When the aura is this colour blue throughout, the emotional health of the subject is at its most positive. It's about communication, learning, calm and peaceful disposition, emotional health, faith and trust, inner voice certainty, clarity, integrity, creativity. On the negative side it can turn to melancholy, immaturity, obsessiveness and spiritual arrogance. Blue can however be contaminated by other colours. For example, blue tinged with grey represents selfish religious feeling. As a general point, for the greatest effect from a colour, it should cover the whole body.

Green shows good affinity between body and soul, a colour of varied significance. Its root meaning is empathy, the act of placing oneself in the position of another person. In its lower aspects it represents deceit and jealousy; higher up in the emotional scale it signifies adaptability and at its very highest when it represents the colour of foliage, sympathy – the very essence of feeling for other people. In its neutral aspects it represents manifestation – taking what we need from the earth to supply our needs. In some shades, green merging into yellow stands for the lower intellectual and critical faculties. Green is associated with healing and teaching energy, renewal or change, magnetism, abundance, calm. In its negative form physical discomfort, deception, distrust or doubt, naivety.

Yellow is an intellectual colour. Each shade of yellow indicates the level of mental functioning. Yellow in general is associated with intellect and intelligence, personal power, scientific mindedness, independence, ingenuity, mental agility, self-starter. The negative aspects include controlling, judging, perfectionism, stubbornness, anxiety or worry.

Bright yellow indicates highest intellect; yellow tinged with red is strong intellect, yellow mixed with an equal part of red indicates a low type of intellect. Many people have a great potential which they do not use. Many go through the motions of work, which has long ceased to be a challenge to them, and are too exhausted to seek intellectual stimulation through an active and varied social life. It is a great tragedy that the sense of the community is diminishing in Western society as large cities crumble from within. Individualism and community support are antithetical in practise. Community spirit is to be found in much greater abundance in smaller, less mobile communities and in so-called primitive society.

Orange is a mixture of red (the physical) and yellow (the mental). It is to do with the generation of activity and is a common attribute of the aura. It is the colour of transition as the subject tries to file information into manageable and balanced units. If the colour remains constant over a period of time it means that the individual is stuck, unable to develop. Muddiness represents lack of clarity or repression of problems. Positive associations are artistic creativity, compassion, sensitivity, harmonizing, healing. Negative qualities involve uncertainty, impressionability, naivety.

Red is the colour of activity. It is the animal element and relates to materialistic thinking. Although it sometimes shows vitality and health on the physical plane it is more likely to show a negative trait. On the mental plane, red indicates anger and its relative pride. Rose red means pure affection; brilliant red implies anger with force; dirty red shows passion and sensuality; brown red reveals avarice. Red is sometimes used in bars and will cause customers to drink more and stimulate base feelings.

Pink is a combination of the active red with the addition of white light. It stands for universal love and is the colour of the heart chakra. It is excellent for taming violent behaviour and to soothe mental disruptions. Some other positive qualities include activity or movement, passion, sexuality, masculine energy, leadership qualities, strong will, vitality, motivation, generosity. Other negative qualities include a forceful or stubborn nature, anger, rage, fear.

Brown is an uncommon colour in the aura, and is often seen as a muddying effect with another colour. Brown can be an affinity with the earth and can show industriousness with agriculture. Normally though, brown indicates depression, or a materialistic, selfish personality. Very frequently, clients who are very open, and quite spiritual themselves, take on the depression of others. When clients say that moods come on them 'for no reason' this is a sign that the origin does not lie in themselves. This transported condition can be seen as a darker cloud which drifts around and is not anchored at one point.

Black is the lack of light. Black absorbs all colour and reflects none. When we talk about 'black clouds of depression' we talk about an area where light has been eliminated, a type of Black Hole. This colour is often linked with malice. Black is frequently found in people who are angry at someone else, for example an ex-wife or husband, and they have allowed their anger to eat into them. They imagine how much they could hurt another person or take revenge for something done to them. Malice (from the Latin *malus* – bad) means to cherish vindictive feelings against, which in many cases becomes a controlling part of the personality. Black is difficult to see; most people just feel it as a force of unease, or of cold. In religious history, black is associated with ignorance and evil. Such people have limited power to remove themselves from the condition they are in because they chose it via their own free will.

Colours can change. Nothing is fixed. Anyone can change anything if they so wish. However, the more you are bound by selfish thoughts the less likely you are to want to change or indeed see the need for change.

IS THE PERCEPTION OF COLOUR NECESSARY?

No, it is not necessary but certainly helpful. The level, volatility or disposition of the aura reflects partly in colour but the regularity of colour effects are just as important. According to clairvoyants, the colours can change from moment to moment and usually vary with mood swings. There is however, no independent scientific corroboration or a method of measuring the wavelength differentials especially as the body radiations are in three- dimensions.

Moreover, also if we see an aura through our own energy field, it is likely to be distorted by our own predispositions.

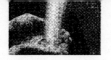

CHAPTER FIVE

METHODS OF READING THE AURA

How does the aura as seen by sensitives correspond with photographic images? First, let us re-examine the validity of photographic methods. Film sensitivity encompasses what we call the 'visible spectrum'. Roughly speaking, this is a wavelength of light from infrared to ultraviolet and includes all the colours of the rainbow. The problem is that under normal film conditions, the very weak light of the aura cannot be detected. Although it is there, the camera responds to average light sensitivity so the aura light is swamped by the background light.

However, not all energies fall into this category. On frequent occasions, ghosts, technically known as 'spirit extras' have been photographed. Whether we define this as an aura is an arguable point. A feature of ghost photography is that the operator cannot see the outline when he takes the picture. It cannot be produced to order. It appears and disappears at will and is most likely a projection of the thought fields of the discarnate person. A discussion about this is outside the scope of this volume and readers are referred to specialist books on the topic.

GENERAL PROBLEMS OF APPROACH

Since the aura is a three-dimensional phenomenon emerging from within the physical body and is very subtle in its patterns, no single process can capture the whole effect. The whole aura shimmers, though its basic nature stays constant unless some drastic event occurs. When you make a Kirlian energy photo it is like one frame from a film. Despite this, the accuracy of the information gained can be quite remarkable. The most helpful plan is to see the aura itself like wind. You cannot see the wind but you can see its effect on the bending of the branches of trees. It is good diagnostic practice never to rely on one method alone. If an aura photograph can give us even one reliable clue, it is worth the effort. The result should be placed alongside the results of other methods for an accurate interpretation.

HOW CAN THE AURA BE PHOTOGRAPHED?

One method is Kirlian photography, or electrophotography. This is a way of recording on film or paper the energy patterns around the hands and feet of human subjects.

It was publicized by Semyon and Valentina Kirlian in 1939 when they noticed that sparks placed in the path of a piece of photosensitive material produced an image. Kirlian called his method 'High frequency, high voltage photography'.

The electrical fields around a body change before any physical disease becomes apparent. The benefits of using Kirlian for medical diagnosis as in cancer screening is that the method is comparatively non-invasive and gives a very early indication with high reliability even from a single sample.

Scientists have made many studies of the force fields around the human body.

Their conclusions are that:
1. The human body has an electrical aspect, part of which is reflected in a 'field' effect not only within it but at a distance from it.
2. This electrical matrix is affected by the physical and mental state of the subject and changes accordingly.
3. The characteristics can be measured by standard electrical measuring apparatus including high impedance volt-meters.
4. The human body radiates light, which varies according to the psychological and physical condition of the body.
5. If the body is placed within the ambit of a high-frequency field and a sheet of photosensitive material is interposed, various patterns are obtained which may be due to a combination of the physical, mental and psychological state of the subject.

These are some of the applications that Kirlian photography has been used for:
1. To measure the life-force in seeds and plants.
2. To detect illness before physical symptoms appear.
3. To cross-check with other therapies such as acupuncture, homoeopathy and spiritual healing.
4. To investigate the residual toxic effects of drug addiction.
5. To evaluate the effect of parental conflict on children.
6. To assess psychological compatibility between two people.

Kirlian has been written about in over 700 scientific papers and I would refer the reader to my book 'The Unseen Self – Kirlian Photography Explained' C.W. Daniel 1997.

ARE THERE OTHER METHODS OF PHOTOGRAPHING THE AURA?

A method known as aura imaging photography claims to photograph the light around a person's head, with a specially adapted Polaroid camera. The subject places their hands in a metal 'glove' and electrodes measure the difference in voltage. They then sit in front of the camera and an exposure is made. On the image of the head, colours are projected. The actual colours, their positions and extent, tell something about their mental and physical condition.

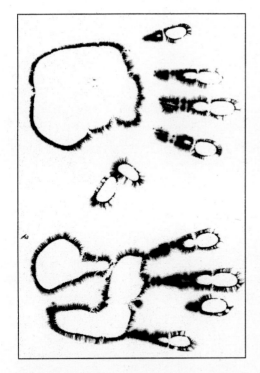

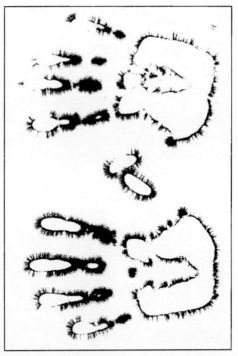

'NO CONFIDENCE' HAND *A man in his 20s – very shy – living reluctantly with his parents. Has difficulty expressing himself. The home environment difficult for his work as an artist.*
NOTE: *'Colourless' appearance indicates lack of spontaneity and ability to relate. Subject needs counselling and support. The left hand (intuition and feeling) is even less radiant than the right hand (logic).*

'UNDER-UTILIZED' HAND *A man in his 30s recently made redundant from the computer industry. Well paid job but understretched. Polarity therapist. Knows he has a lot of discovering to do.*
NOTE: *'Plenty of energy reservoirs (black areas down fingers). Left hand stronger than right hand. Also note inner band round fingertips which is a sign of strength of personality.*

Another method, known as the Polycontrast Interface Photography (PIP) system enables a multicoloured image of the body to be seen on video or still photographs. A patient is placed against a white background with a full spectrum, fluorescent light above the head.

A video camera filled with a CCD (a semi-conducting device) is focused on the subject. The CCD has light-sensitive cells which transform light into electrical signals. These electrical signals are fed into a specially developed computer programme which assigns each signal with a number, according to its intensity. These numbers relate to a particular colour, or shade of colour.

Finally the image of the patient is displayed on the screen, as a multi-coloured image with the energy centres, meridians and problem areas clearly visible according to the light patterns in each area.

The promoters claim that the body's energy fields are being revealed, and that the effects of healing can be shown. Healthy areas of the body show up as yellow, green or blue, whilst red coloration suggests congestion. The method can show the balancing effect of crystal healing, to give but one example.

HOW DO THESE METHODS OF PHOTOGRAPHING COMPARE?

Let us look at what the four methods achieve.

1. Clairvoyance or sensitive observation

Clairvoyants or sensitives work subjectively. They see a band of colour around the subject with layers, shape and intensity. Just as important, they feel impressions coming from the subject. This will be partly received with the 'inner eye', partly with extended vision and partly with the nervous system. The disadvantage is that an evaluation is more difficult to verify and is not quite so susceptible to scientific investigation. This brings up the interesting question of verifying psychic phenomena which we will discuss later.

The other three methods are independent of the operator. This means that the results are there for all to see, and meaning is subject to interpretation by the diagnostician. Subjective evaluation does enter into the equation but only to a small extent. However, it should be born in mind that in all experiments with subtle energy, the state of mind of the operator or the observer can influence the subject directly.

2. The Kirlian photograph

Some observers regard Kirlian as rather limited because it is not possible to observe the whole body at once. It lends itself to flat surfaces such as hands and feet. From the practical point of view this is not such a handicap as you might think, since the richness of nervous tissue and the formative influences of palmistry, acupuncture and reflexology ensure an interesting result. Kirlian, then, produces a 'slice' of the aura from which the condition of the whole aura can be deduced. It is not, however, possible to see the effect of healing whilst it is happening. There are specialist machines where you can put your hand on a glass plate and see the change in radiations. The problem is that what you see with your eye is not what the film or paper sees – a misleading impression can be gained.

The Kirlian photograph can be used as a valuable diagnostic aid, but it is even more valuable when a photograph is made before and after an intervention or counselling. The effectiveness of the intervention can be easily seen. Unlike the impact of the reports by the clairvoyant, there is an observed therapeutic effect of the sight of the Kirlian photo on the subject.

3. The Aura Imaging photograph

This method consists of the superimposition of various images on a Polaroid film. Some may consider this method misleading in that the aura that the camera sees is not around the head. The colours are simply projected on to the head. The aura imaging photograph may well offer us circumstantial evidence about the condition of the person, but the colours themselves only show us the result of a condition, not the cause of it.

4. Polycontrast Interface Photography (PIP)

The contribution made by the PIP may well be the most interesting. The method is non-invasive. This means that it does not interfere with the subject whilst the method is in progress, as the camera is at a distance and the subject is asked to assume a passive role. This would make the method suitable for evaluating the effect of the healer on the colour and balance of the energy field.

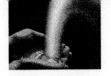

CHAPTER SIX

BUILDING AND STRENGTHENING THE AURA

Human beings are deep wells of energy, immense reservoirs of force, but the real problem (of energy blocks) has not changed one bit through the ages. The question must include enquiries about the nature of our priorities? Do we want to invest our energy and attention in making a successful material life for ourselves and our family for security's sake, or do we want to throw ourselves and our whole being into the fire of spiritual life? Most people are too lethargic even to pose this fundamental question seriously. Many remain dilettantes, dabblers in spiritual life.

In order to build and strengthen the aura, the first task is to acknowledge that the aura exists, the second is to become aware of the detail, the third is to find the willpower to change. The rules of the auric bodies are different. The physical body is an intrinsic part of our existence and needs to be maintained by nutrition and exercise. The other bodies must also be developed through a conscious process of internal evolution. Commitment and effort is required to achieve the phasing in, full expression and liberation of these bodies. The physical body and the mind are the co-founders of the subtle body, and the subtle body as it develops becomes the foundation for the cosmic body.

It is therefore confusing why some people choose to starve and otherwise negate the physical body in order to advance spiritual development. Others starve in order to cleanse from impurities. The body is the temple of the soul, as Jesus said. Whilst incarnated, we need our body and it should be esteemed and treated with respect. The idea is to transcend the limitations of the body. Nothing is evil. We may eat and drink to the maximum yet if our other bodies are undernourished, we will not be satisfied. The question is how to activate the subtle bodies. We need to use the physical body, the mind, the rationale, features of the physical environment, not ignore them. They are tools. They are the means.

With regard to colour, it is interesting that light and colour itself has been used to strengthen the aura. The therapeutic use of sunlight and colours – heliotherapy – is as old as medicine itself. Egyptian physicians used rooms with coloured walls to heal various afflictions.

Sun baths became very popular in the late 19th-century Germany within the framework of the naturopathy movement. Ultraviolet light therapy was founded as a result of the discoveries by Koch and Pasteur on the role of bacteria in illness. Light has been used to treat scarring after chicken-pox, tuberculosis, rickets, some skin diseases and the healing of wounds.

Another way is to use music. Music may not only be the food of love, it may also help to keep infections at bay and to improve the tone of the aura. Dr. Francis Brannaf, assistant professor at Wilkes University in Pennsylvania has commented on how little research has been done on how levels of immunoglobulin (IgA) are affected by the positive feelings induced by music. Stress affects the immune system and decreases the immuno- efficiency so that people get sick at times of stress – during exams, bereavement, divorce and so on. IgA is a front-line antibody carried in the saliva and mucous. It responds rapidly to viral attack and when levels are low, people are more vulnerable and more likely to become infected. Dr. Brannaf and his fellow researcher Prof. Carl Charnetski exposed people to a range of stimuli including elevator 'musak', jazz music, silences, tone noises and clicks. They found that after 30 minutes of exposure to musak, the antibody levels in the saliva of the listeners had increased by 14%. When they played jazz, with interruptions for traffic reports and news items, the IgA had gone up by only half as much, about 7%. Silence had no effect, but when the subjects were exposed to annoying sounds such as clicking, IgA levels plummetted by 20%.

We have already seen that the aura has two functions: to inform and to protect. Our aura can work for us and against us. We can draw good luck or ill fortune. This decision is ours and ours alone. That is the nature of free will. No therapeutic method can be considered healthy if it does not place the responsibility of self healing at the feet of the client. We have made our bed, and so we must lie on it, as the phrase goes.

THE RELATIONSHIP BETWEEN HEALING AND DIAGNOSIS

An act of understanding on the part of the sensitive therapist and the subject must constitute an act of healing. A breakthrough in understanding will be the catalyst that can cause increased balance between the constituent parts of the body. Let's look a little at the nature of the body and the mechanism of healing. All living objects give out fields. Some are electromagnetic. This means they have qualities of electricity and magnetism in them. All living things emit light and this we have called the aura. It is only a matter of time before computer analysis will be able to offer instant diagnosis of illness but meanwhile we should examine the properties of the human being as a healer. No human being, no cell can exist without feed-back. The quickest way of creating madness is to put someone in a room deprived of any sort of stimulus.

As we have a mind, body, soul and spirit, the methods below are based on this assumption. All must be taken into consideration. It is no good feeding your body with the correct food when the mind is languishing for stimulus or the soul is troubled with conscience about some unresolved matter.

The general approaches are:

The mind – thinking

1. Increasing understanding about ourselves
2. Facing any factor that is troubling us

The body – surviving

1. Treating our body correctly and providing the correct nutrition
2. Exercising and resting it and using correct breathing

The soul – being

1. Finding a faith which makes sense and carries us forward
2. Mixing in fellowship with others

The spirit – living

1. Disciplining ourselves as if preparing for a race. Setting daily targets. Making realistic goals and objectives.

The general approach to a problem of any nature is:

1. assessment – distinguishing the original cause from the presenting problem
2. clearing – separating the emotional feelings from the material facts
3. counselling through listening, sharing, being a catalyst
4. support services after the sessions have concluded

There are many ways to obtain information from the client, the sensing of colour being one. These depend on the accurate perception of the aura for their effectiveness. An effective method deals not only with the symptoms but works on all levels with all the complexities and disharmonies that create disease. One of these treatments is 'Aura Soma'. The name is derived from the Greek word 'Soma' meaning 'body' or 'living energy' in Sanscrit. It is based on the need to restore balance between mind, body and spirit and thus enable the body to resume its normal rhythm.

Many of us know subconsciously what our problems are and what we need. In the Aura Soma method, colour is the key that gives access to our ability to know what is right and true for us. This 'self-selective' ability works when subjects are asked to pick in order of attractiveness bottles that are shown to them. The first bottle shows our task for life; the second is the way that the task is taken up, the third is the 'now' and the fourth is the future influences impinging on us. The bottles contain various mixtures of emulsified essential oils and aroma essences with water-based solutions of herb and flower extracts and gem essences. A consultation is based upon a selection of four balance bottles. The choice by the client provides the key to unlock the difficulties of the past and confirm gifts and strengths. A consultation interprets the messages of the colours, exploring with clients their healing journey.

There are two types of oils 'Pomanders' and 'Quintessences'. Pomanders are designed primarily to give auric protection, acting specifically on the electromagnetic field which closely surrounds the physical body. They also strengthen and repair the energetic field. The aura is reinforced with the vibration of the colour needed and acts as a protection, enabling the retention of etheric integrity. Pomander drops are placed in the left palm; the hands are rubbed together and then held out in a gesture which offers the energy to the world as well as to ourselves. The hands are then passed around the aura from top to bottom, as if one were gently stroking the electromagnetic field an inch or two away from the physical body. Correct breathing allows the absorption of the energies through the mucous membranes.

Quintessences are subtle in their effect and help us to align ourselves with a particular quality of energy, to open ourselves to receive energetic assistance for a particular project. Fine movements of the hands round the body stimulate and draw down these subtle energies.

PSYCHIC PROTECTION

The word protection comes from the Latin *tegere*, to cover. There is a big trap in this. If there is disharmony within the psyche the inner weakness will resonate with the external force and techniques will be unproductive. Excessive optimism about the human condition – much loved by more expansive psychologies found in North America – is of limited use. Protection comes about automatically and is proportionate to the amount of integratory work that has been achieved. It is not true that protection is in proportion to the desire to be so, or the amount of knowledge. It is the state of innocence which protects. If we naturally radiate love and light, then no evil can touch us. Others would say that it is being fully 'grounded' in your body – phantasy thinkers and dreamers will never be fully secure.

However, given that work is ongoing, are there any procedures or rituals that we can use in our everyday lives? A positive and productive life is the first requirement. Laziness and spiritual torpor are not helpful. Any matter that causes worry should be quickly dealt with. 'Never let the sun set on your anger' is a good motto.

A few simple ideas include imagining ourselves enclosed from top to toe in a bubble of light. This will give us all-round protection. Imagine a fine filter which allows out and receives fine vibrations. Remember that each 'bubble' is unique and should contain symbols of what we believe in – for the Christian, a cross, for the Hindu, the AUM sign. This discipline should be practised every day until thinking in these terms is instinctive.

In addition to the bubble, you can try imagining a shield or mirror of light. This will bounce back and return any negative thoughts from other people. If you feel that someone has bad social attitudes then cover the area of the solar plexus in your own aura. In the case of attack that has been partly successful, have a shower and allow the water to run down your spine. This is particularly helpful for healers who have seen 'difficult' clients. Remember that when the feeling of depletion reaches the conscious mind, the damage has already been done. After all healing or counselling sessions have a ritual shower or cleansing exercise as a matter of discipline, whether you feel you need it or not.

In addition there are many crystals and minerals which can help us on the physical and psychic planes. For example Amber purifies and draws out negative energies and cleanses the atmosphere of negative vibrations. Black tourmaline deflects negative and psychic energies and assists with grounding. Jasper induces deep tranquillity and relaxation, Rose quartz opens the heart chakra and brings about the actuality of universal love. Specialist literature will assist you to find the crystal or mineral that is right for you, or learn to use your own intuition.

Protection does not come about from one single event of intent. Attention to detail will bring about a cumulative effect slowly but surely. The regular cleansing and protection of the home or office should not be neglected. Any metal object introduced into the home, or any crystal, will have its own charge, good or bad. Apart from general cleanliness, specific flowers can be used to maintain the purity of your home. For example, roses absorb negative vibrations. The white rose, a powerful symbol of purity, absorbs the most. Carnations are good for sick-rooms and the calming of mental and emotional turmoil. Small rituals such as lighting a candle for peace every day can create a safe and harmonious energy. When you leave a home for a period of time, making the sign of a cross or using a revered symbol can bolster safety. This should be performed by all entrances and windows and in the centre of the room.

Obsessive or paranoid states of mind will ensure that you are more open to negative influences and psychic forces of all kinds. By contrast, a light and happy disposition will create a most unattractive environment for such influences!

Excessive worry can often be a barrier to any breakthrough. Many of my clients come in such a wound-up state that they are unable to listen to any advice. The problem is that the person is too sensitive for their own good and in this case any psychic gift is difficult to handle. De-focusing from all psychic perceptions gives the client a chance to figure out what they have experienced, and recover from emotional surprise or shock. This helps them to return to normal reality if they are feeling too disorientated.

How do we rebalance our psychology? Traditional psychology is concerned with and is an authority on 'endarkenment'. Look at any psychology directory to find abreaction, neurosis, withdrawal, conflict, aggression. Esoteric knowledge is concerned with 'enlightenment'. It's a textbook of 'how to grow'.

We cannot accomplish this by any quick fix method or by any special ambition. Rather, we need to remove all desire and all pretentiousness by working from the base upwards. We can achieve this over a period of time by relaxing and focusing all conscious thought toward the physical world and down-to-earth activity, seeing it for what it is – and what it is not. There are several approaches that help with this. Becoming involved with other people, preferably with a lot of social interaction and discussion. Engage in physical activity; walk around, stretch, jog, or do anything else that makes you more aware of your physical body. Let the thoughts of the psychic experiences float away like a dream, without worrying about them. If there is anything you especially enjoy doing, like games, programming, writing, art, etc., involve yourself deeply in that. Do anything you can think of to keep your mind and body occupied together in the physical world, and don't let memories distract you from it. When you are ready to restart (and move out of shut down), simply start opening your perceptions again as you would when you first practice any psychic ability. You can do this at any time, whenever you are comfortable and ready to do it.

Under normal circumstances, a shield will maintain itself for quite a while before becoming depleted. However, such factors as large amounts of negative thinking, illness, and lack of sleep can all cause a weak shield. This section details how to maintain a shield more successfully under stressful conditions.

The most common difficulty in maintaining the integrity of our aura is daily stress. While a shield often helps prevent psychic energy from adding to the stress, eventually the shield can weaken. The best cure is more rest, planned time alone and meditating, and noticing what environmental factors are stressful, and avoiding them. Regular meditation helps a lot to replenish drained energy, and it also helps relieve the internal stress that weakens the shield.

Empathic overload is similar, but can be more intense than normal stress. As many empaths have realized, large crowds, schools, and cities are often filled with intense emotional energy. Empaths who are particularly sensitive to this learn to build very strong shields to keep other people's emotions separate from impinging on their own. The first few days of an emotionally intense environment can be particularly wearing if the empath has not yet made a strong enough shield. To protect from the empathic pounding of emotionally charged environments, meditation and careful examination of the self are very important. Meditation helps relieve the stress and emotional energy in a controlled way. It also gives time to identify the difference between empathic emotions and personal emotions. By identifying the self carefully (especially emotionally), an extra layer is added to the shield defining 'own emotions' and 'external emotions' and separating the two. This helps greatly in making external emotions bounce off harmlessly.

Occasionally, electromagnetic fields can tear at a shield, causing it to weaken. This happens most commonly in people who work with high power electronic equipment or who live near large power lines. If the person has grown up in those conditions, the shield will probably already be adjusted to take that into account. For people who have just dropped in to that environment, though, it can be a rather intense pounding. In this case, careful examination of the electromagnetic field energies and personal shield energies can help the shield adjust. Experiment with drawing energy from the field and transmuting it into a more useful form of energy. With some conscious practice, getting the shield to adjust to that energy takes only a little effort.

Taking part in psychic 'confrontations' is the another area where shields become weakened. Though this is an area that most people will not ever need to deal with, there are some who can't avoid it (and may have known they were dealing with it before ever picking up a book on psychic abilities). Shielding is a natural defense; it can become weakened when attacked too strongly. During psychic battle, shields are held in place strongly by will power and energy. Will power has the most control over the shield. Total confidence in the self (not arrogance, but confidence to stay in place and not be budged) is the best way to keep a shield from being drained. If it does start being drained, drawing energy through a comfortable source to add to it will help replenish it. Basically, keep drawing and don't let up until you know you are no longer in danger. If you feel you can not hold up the strength any longer, consider placing your psychic self some place safe (or even shutting down) to avoid actually being attacked. Attack rarely causes any physical manifestation stronger than a headache, but headaches can get pretty bad. Avoidance is best.

Empathy is the ability to feel someone else's emotions. It is the most common of all psychic abilities, and often people have it without fully realizing it. It sometimes shows up as someone feeling a friend is hurt or in trouble, without being physically present. Empathy also shows as someone being stressed because a friend is, without having any apparent reason to be stressed themselves.

An empathic connection can be created by focusing on the person you want to connect with. Use a similar focus to that of projecting, but rather than travelling to the person, feel energy connecting you to them. Let it grow and strengthen, as webs or joined hands holding you together. Emotions flow through it, either in one direction or both, depending on what you want. Open up to receive images through the link. You may feel the emotions as if they were your own, or you may feel slightly distanced from them. They may appear as emotionally charged images, or merely as gut feelings. You will probably become familiar with their form very quickly after opening a link.

As you receive images, watch for related details. Notice any subtler feelings associated with what you are receiving. Practice navigating between various areas of feelings by feeling your way through the related emotions. Controlled navigation can take a while to learn, but it is necessary for choosing what you receive and eventually learning telepathy.

Closing a link is just as important as opening it. When you are ready to close a link, visualize it gently drawing apart and closing off. If you try to simply remove it, it may hurt like a suddenly broken relationship. It could even hurt physically near the heart (which is where empathy typically connects). Be gentle with empathic links, because they are representative of your relationship with the person on the other end. Both people are affected by it, in good and bad ways. Watching the natural empathic links between people can tell you a lot about how they interact. (This, of course, does take practice though.)

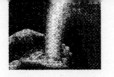

PART TWO

THE CHAKRAS

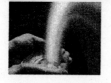

CHAPTER SEVEN

THE NATURE OF THE CHAKRAS

A chakra is circular in its dynamic, having a specific centre. It is situated within the body, not as a part of the gross body but as a supramaterial power form. It is imprinted in the body and is undetectable by normal scientific methodology. Because of its subtle character a chakra is not seen with the eyes, even with the help of supersensitive instruments, though resulting colours can be seen with the inner eye. Some scientists, notably Dr Hiroshi Motoyama have claimed to detect chakras by sensitive scanning devises but these results are more likely to indicate electrical fields of the nerve plexuses associated with each chakra rather than the chakras themselves.

The word chakra is Sanskrit for wheel or circle, and these vortices have a circular, whirling appearance as they draw various forces and energies into the body. Each of them is depicted in a variety of ways, using deities, colours, symbols and letters to represent various qualities and energies. Most commonly, the shape of the flower is used as a symbolic expression of the ability of a chakra to unfold like a flower. The Rosicrucians used the Rose Cross to depict man and his chakras; each rose on the cross identified a chakra in the subtle body. In India the lotus has been used as a symbol of the chakras. They are often referred to as lotuses. The lotus is a flower that has its roots in the mud (material world), its stem grows up through the water (the astral or emotional world), and the bloom rising above the water into the air (the realm of the mind).

C G Jung, described the chakras as gateways of consciousness in humankind, receptive points for the inflow of energies from the cosmos to the spirit and soul of man. Chakras are not spiritual in themselves. They are simply part of the invisible body. Of course there is a sense that the whole world is spiritual, but the chakras in particular and the aura in general are ethically and spiritually neutral. The condition of the chakras are simply expressions of equilibrium or otherwise of the subtle body of man. These vortexes can be perceived as spinning cones of energy. They are centred in the spine not in the fatty tissue in the front.

In order to nourish us physically, emotionally, mentally and spiritually, the chakras take in energy from the universal field which exists all around us. Due to the power of our own constitution, however, they also radiate (or re-radiate) energy. Chakras can be seen as computers, seven large ones surrounded by a number of smaller interdependent ones. Each one is programmed to interpret our reality. Mental and physical illness occurs when different chakras give and receive contradictory messages and patterns. Unfortunately, this understanding is a prohibited area to a doctor of Western medicine.

We have seen the nature and complexity of our chemical processes. In addition to the circulation of blood, and the existence of millions of nerves, Chinese medicine describes many thousands of major paths and combinations of paths – the acupuncture meridians and nadis. The nadis, it is claimed, send electricity through the body, and millions of small pathways transport varying amounts of energy.

WHY SHOULD WE TAKE AN INTEREST IN OUR CHAKRAS?

Our normal form of awareness is essentially physical. We are so conditioned by current systems of belief and ethics that we forget that there are other natural ways of seeing which complement the mechanistic belief that our mind constructs from the chemical and physiological reactions in our physical brain. It is a pity that we have to counterpoise the scientist and the mystic's approach but alas the two world views are still diametrically opposed. This guarantees that debate will continue for a very long time!

We all know the practical helplessness of a person who cannot boil an egg or mend a fuse or does not know what goes on under the bonnet of their car. These are illustrations of incapability in the physical world. Incompetence in the spiritual world is just as forbidding. If our energies are 'us' and play a vital part in the quality of life then in order to function in this world we need to understand ourselves. The spine is considered the main axis around which the electromagnetic energy field forms. The north pole of the human energy field is located in the brain ventricle, the south pole at the base of the spine.

If there is harmony between mind, body, soul and spirit the energy paths run parallel, inducing and reinforcing each other. The various currents of energy must be in harmony both with each other and with the universe. When this is achieved, the person is at peace with the universe and he or she will naturally draw towards them those people, situations, and karma which are necessary for self-development.

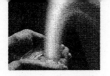

The seven major Chakras discussed

There are seven major chakras dealing with various aspects and levels of consciousness. Before we discuss them it should be emphasized that no chakra is 'better' than another. We would not say that the engine of a car is more important than the wheels! All the chakras need to work in harmony. Without the lower chakras we could not live effectively in this world. The key thing is our creative use and understanding of them.

The functions of the major chakras

The first chakra is the root or *Muladhara* chakra located at the perineum which is mid-way between the anus and the genitals. It has four petals, the colours of which vary according to different schools of thought. They are a shining red and gold, yellow or golden, or red like the jawa flower. The chakra externalizes as the adrenal glands and governs the spine and kidneys. It also influences all the cells of the body. This represents the physical body and the demands of the physical world – in a word – survival. It encompasses the most fundamental operations of physical maintenance and overall wellbeing. We speak of getting to the root of the problem. In other words, let's see the true chain of cause and effect.

The two lowest chakras are both connected with our sexuality and unconscious motivations. Once again we find that the pineal gland is intimately connected with all aspects of sexual functioning, both in terms of reproduction and secondary sexual aspects. The physical functioning mirrors the yogic lore.

On a psychological level, this root chakra is about becoming incarnated. Before we can become embodied in flesh we need to accept our situation and then become grounded or rooted. That is why early experiences of playing as a child are so important. Playing assists conceptual thought and in later life our relationships and social functioning. Associated with this chakra are various negative psychological states. We can find stress, anxiety, insecurity or hyperactivity. On the positive side, we can find calmness and the ability to remove tension, and become energetic and strong.

The second chakra, located level with the coccyx is termed the *Svadisthana* or sacral chakra. It is connected with sexual and reproductive life and is the intimate

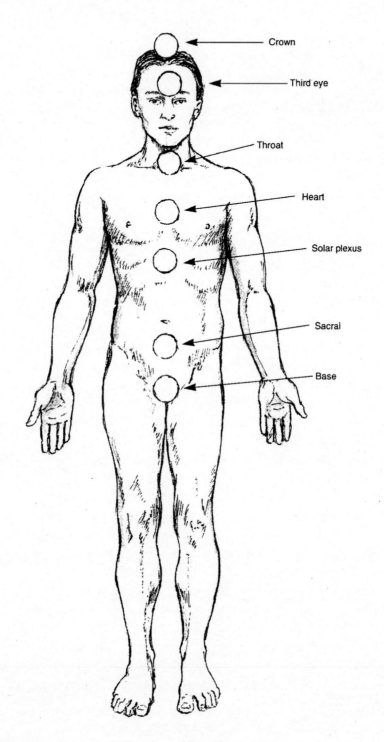

Crown

Third eye

Throat

Heart

Solar plexus

Sacral

Base

THE SEVEN MAJOR CHAKRAS

and totally personal aspect of being. In this modern world this is the chakra that is most frequently abused. Whilst open, deep relationships and connections are possible. Whilst closed, feelings and sexuality remain disconnected. The closed chakra is a barrier, a closed door to sharing, intimacy and the true invitation to know another person. This chakra is not about sexual encounter as such but in the exchange of intimacy and the sharing of subtle energies which enrich and nourish. Negative psychological states are frustration, anger, aggression, poor self-esteem, suppression of sexual energy, emotional blockages, depression. Positively we find creativity, initiative, integration of emotions, ability to feel intimacy with others.

The third chakra is termed the *Manipuraor*, or solar plexus. The word can be translated as 'city of jewels' or 'filled with jewels'. It is the centre of all our sentiments and emotions and contributes towards the value of life. We express ourselves in laughter and crying – a thing which animals cannot do. The tendency for modern man to repress emotions and to pretend to be perfect prevents the development of this centre. The correctly adjusted centre provides an easy alliance between thinking and feeling. Negative states are grief, depression, emotional problems and disturbances, inability to remove stress. Positive states are the ability to balance emotions and thus emotional wellbeing; emotional security.

At the solar plexus we have the adrenals, the fight or flight hormones connected with fear, short-term stress, 'gut reactions' and digestion. The adrenals' function is intimately connected with the pineal gland in many ways at a physiological level, and this physical function closely mirrors the teaching of the yogis about the solar plexus centre.

These three chakras comprise our interface with physical living. In order for us to be able to reach the higher levels of awareness, there must be harmony between these three. We need to be aware of our gross material body, because if we cannot do this, then we cannot be aware of our invisible subtle body. In the course of a day we should not function like automatons but recognize and respect the function of our physical body to support our life and enable our soul to go forward on its journey. Likewise, if we remain fixed and focused on our physical body and its needs then as a human being we remain asleep. This body is not an end in itself but just the means to an end. As Jesus said "the body is the temple of the spirit".

Emotions such as anger need to be recognized. Anger is born in the mind but manifests in the physical body. Glands secrete hormones. The rate of the heart beat increases. So we have anger itself, and then the manifestation of anger. We can try and control the symptoms. This is known as repression, but unfortunately the source of anger remains and will contaminate the other chakras. We often become aware of the existence of love, fear or anger when they have reached an advanced stage – and sometimes only when we have expressed our emotions in the outside world. An act of aggression starts in our etheric body and it is a mark of the developed person that they use their sensitivity to detect a shrinking or distortion of this creator of emotions before it manifests. If we live in the conditions that make the etheric body clear, then harmony will more likely follow. If we live in conditions that make the body distort, then disharmony will prevail. Eventually this will create a prison from which the individual will find it hard to escape.

The fourth chakra is the *Anahata* chakra. It is the centre of the heart. The heart is in the middle; three centres above and three below. It symbolizes the interface between materialism and spirituality or the door between the lower consciousness and the higher consciousness. The heart is the centre of the soundless 'sound'. In the heart there is no word – it is wordless.

The heart is not physical. It is the place from which love arises. It is not senti-mental. Sentiments are momentary. In the modern Western world, sentiment and love are confused. Love is a capacity. Sentiment is a sensation – like eating ice cream. The wordless dialogue of heart to heart communication is timeless and non-linguistic. It is worth making the effort to look at the symbolism of the heart since in almost every spiritual belief system great emphasis is placed on it together with the power of love itself. Great teachers and philosophers have stated that we are here on this planet mainly to learn how to love and transform our experiences with the transforming power of our love.

The acts of loving – and forgiving – ourselves and others have the most profound effect upon our life; our physical health, our emotional and mental state, and our spirituality. The heart is indeed a crucible, an instrument of conversion, capable of evincing a compassion for the human condition, metabolizing the energy that moves through it into a new and higher frequency. This higher frequency energy equates with a higher consciousness. This is why the heart chakra is called the bridge between the lower three chakras, whose energies are concerned with how to live in the world of matter, and the upper three chakras, whose energies have a higher vibration and deal with the world of spirit.

If the heart chakra is closed or unbalanced, the energy of an event continuously recycles itself through our lower three chakras. We sometimes begin to relish the negative energy generated by an event. It may bring us power over people, sympathy from them, or may allow us to continuously discharge anger in various inappropriate ways. With the heart closed, we have no access to our 'forgiving energy', and we make a choice, consciously or unconsciously, to refuse to let go of the hurtful events. Consequently, there is no resolution; the experience remains in our energy fields, and in our lives, as unfinished business. The energies of our lower three chakras are re-routed into the negative belief systems triggered by the event. Sending our energy into negative belief systems takes it away from our healthy physical body, healthy emotional and mental state, and healthy spirituality.

When we say that we cannot forgive we end up paying for it with our cell tissue, as well as our peace of mind. Conversely, the open heart chakra has a purifying effect upon the energy moving through it, and that energy is then available to move into the upper three chakras.

The fifth, *Vishuddha* or throat chakra, always brings us to an increased awareness of ourselves. The fifth chakra demands that we speak the truth, and part of that truth-speaking is an acknowledgment of our own issues, negative behaviours, and masks to the outer world. Also contained in the throat chakra is the energy of our will. It is symbolized by purity and is the richest, the culmination of human effect – the peak of love, of compassion, of everything that is worthwhile and the door to the zone of egolessness. Already, labour and effort are necessary but they are already becoming redundant. 'Method' or 'technique' cease to be applicable in this chakra. It is the spiritual or etheric body. Any duality between the mind and the spirit ends with the fifth body. The fifth body is non-dual. To develop this realm one only has to enter it. Negative psychological features are introversion, the inability to express oneself and one's feelings, and lack of confidence. Positively, there is a good ability for self-expression and a keen interest in spiritual subjects. Relationships improve because each sees themselves as a source of creativity and does not lean on the other person for support.

In the throat we have the thyroid and parathyroid glands which are concerned with metabolic function and stress. This is the point known by the yogis as Vishuddi, which they connect with immortality. The greater our metabolic rate and the higher and more chronic our stress levels, the sooner our death, so physically the thyroids are connected with life span. These levels are affected by reducing metabolic rate and stress levels.

When the throat chakra speaks the truth, the sixth chakra, also called the third eye or brow or *ajna*, begins to see the truth. On a physical level, the sixth chakra regulates the organs of sight, the eyes; it also has to do with insight, seeing events symbolically, not just in a literal way. The interpretation of events allows us to understand them on a deeper, more unconscious, level. The essence of this modality has little to do with the linear mind, as we begin to understand events from an expanded perspective. It is as if we can step outside our lives, and see that the experiences that come to us are exactly what we need for our growth. We find meaning and insights in our lives. Our job here is to see the situation so clearly, that we empower ourselves and are able, simply by our presence, to comfort and uplift others so that they can then empower themselves.

This chakra is commonly called the 'third eye'. To have mastery of this chakra means that we are masters of our own life, not the slave. It marks the beginning of mysticism and the end of the need for a reliance on religious rituals. We control the flow of information to and from the third eye and the will can be used with clarity and purity. In practise we are subject to the pull and push of desires on the lower plains and very few attain the single-mindedness necessary for mastery. At this level, our will reflects more the divine will than our own ego.

The sixth chakra is linked to the cosmic body. The expression of this is perception, or consciousness. This consciousness is not of 'me'. It is only consciousness – not 'our' existence but only existence. How do we examine the activity of this chakra? This is very difficult with the Western scientific method, though indications can be perceived as individual awareness is eliminated. Those who work within this chakra will begin to recall the vast infinite expanse that is witnessed. This is the viewing point for the infinite, the timeless.

Features to watch out for are a retreat from reality into phantasy. Mental disturbances and problems which arise from indiscriminate reception of unhelpful external thought patterns. Positively, the person has a good ability for creative visualisation, insight, understanding, inspiration, intuition and a clear mind.

The seventh chakra is the crown chakra or *Sahasrara* chakra. It is the ultimate, because now you have crossed even the world of causation. You have gone to the original source. Humankind's methodology can be of little help and indeed mortal factors can be a hindrance. From the point of view of practical life, the journey can be lonely. To enter this realm, a mind without desires or expectations is needed. A mind not longing or desiring or seeking. There are no objects on this plain, only being.

This is the most complete contrast to our normal consciousness which is a shrunken, distorted and contorted version of our cosmic or real consciousness.

The dangers here are an introspection of the higher self and no interest in anything mundane. Positively, there is a sense of fulfilment, of completion, of integration and alignment with God and with higher energies. This is the opening of the 'higher self'.

Sahasrara means 'thousand petalled lotus'. At this level – attained by few – we become this lotus and don't have to go to any other flower for honey – other bees start to come to us from the whole earth and indeed beyond. This is what the eastern mystics call *nirvana*. A person in this level is possessed of intelligence in the way that the top of a maypole is in touch via the strings with all those who hold on at the bottom. It is to do with the ability to bring things together, to summise, to incorporate. With this heightened state, analysis and synthesis takes place instinctively and immediately. There is not the awareness of the passing of time nor the confinement of space. To attain this level is to move from having to being into non-being. Some see this non-being level as a void. It is in fact a state of mind devoid of force, of complexity, of contradiction and it is that level in which all absolutes are confined.

Dwelling within this chakra, our attitude to death is positive, we have the feeling that we know all that is the essence of worthwhileness, we have a feeling of self-value without needing to feel special in the eyes of others; we have a natural feeling of compassion for all other living beings. We do not have to 'try' and be loving – we embody it. So, whereas the mind tends to over-concretize things, the cosmic awareness tends to provide the perfect balance. As St. Paul said, "we can be in the world but not of it."

SPACE AND TIME

What is the relevance of time to all these chakras? Time is supremely relevant in the base chakra as it is irrelevant in the crown chakra. That is the meaning of the word sublimity. It is where there is no time and no space. I suggest that 'hell' is being confined in space and time because our auras are by their nature the free-moving interface between the temporal side of us and our immortal, eternal side. Hence 'heaven' or 'nirvana' is the movement towards the predominance of the higher chakras.

Are there any chakras above this one? Some writers talk of a 'Stellar Gateway' which is located about 12 inches above the top of the head and is the highest chakra that can be incorporated into the human system. This chakra is activated with two essential elements. One is the vitalizing cosmic rays emanating from the great central sun, which our planet and our beings are now receiving. The second critical element required to reignite the Stellar Gateway is the power of the human will focussed in conscious intention. With both of these components present, a human being is capable of spiritually nurturing all aspects of the self by maintaining a direct link to the Divine Impersonal.

Once again let us remind ourselves. Chakras are not in themselves spiritual. They report on the symmetry between our mortal temporal aspects and our eternal, real aspects. Let us say that for all practical purposes there are seven chakras. Within them lie all the means as well as all the barriers to self-fulfilment. Barriers are very useful since these very obstacles when transformed become our means to progress. Where are these barriers? There are no barriers outside therefore there is less need to seek 'outside'. This puts the consumer society in some perspective. Alcohol and drugs, for example, are a subconscious attempt to introduce harmony into the inner regions. This is somewhat like a beggar asking for money when he or she has millions in an untouched bank account. To ignore these riches – available at the behest of our will – is to revert to a status little better than an animal. Dreams we always have – vision has to be developed as a quest and as an evolutionary discipline. It is that quality which marks a developed soul.

WHAT GENERAL FUNCTIONS DO CHAKRAS HAVE?

There are two main activities of the chakras. First they register the harmony of the physical, mental, emotional and spiritual health of the individual.

Secondly, they report on and resonate with chakras of other living beings. Whilst we can respond with all living and non- living things, plants and animals, it is in the human being that the scope for resonance is most complete. It is through and from the chakras that we derive joy and fulfilment from life. It follows that damage to a chakra is one of the most harmful things that can happen to the quality of life.

My own professional work consists of analysing chakras and producing a series of recommendations for the client. Although the interplay between the chakras will always be a mystery, a series of working hypotheses can be produced. Chakras are not just indicators like traffic lights. Each sends out a distinctive energy pattern on a 24 hour basis.

Examining one's own chakras requires a degree of objectivity which most of us do not have and it is preferable that they are examined by another party. My remarks are intended for the person who has started on the path to self-discovery. In order to enter fully into the mode for viewing, we need to base ourselves in an alternate reality state. This involves a predominance in our brain of the alpha wave state, otherwise known as the state of meditation. A non-directive, meditative state is the passport to these other realities. These are said to reside in the right brain. This does not mean that the left brain – the thinking modality – should be numbed – but that both halves should be synchronized. A quiet mind lets go of counter- productive beliefs and habits of body tensions and other malfunctions, allowing the reassertion of normal healthy functioning. In these states, mind, matter and time will have different relationships to everyday sensory reality. Tense people can rarely see auras or do any useful detection work of subtle energies.

THE EFFECT OF DRUGS AND OTHER MEDICATION

The chakras are by their nature subtle in functioning. The nature of allopathic medicine is to reach in from without and adjust the chemical balance in the body together with the suppression of messages that go from the nervous system to the centres of pain.

Drugs can affect the aura a great deal. In my clinical experience I have noted the long-term effects of drug episodes more than 20 years ago. The crown chakra once over-stimulated takes a long time to recover. It tilts off its vertical axis. The individual becomes confused as to their own identity. Drug episodes are felt by me by placing my hand over people's heads as 'pin pricks' or very small disturbances in the aura. These need repair by healing. In many cases, the subject is not even aware of anything untoward.

Sensitives have seen dark energy forms in the liver left over from drugs. Hepatitis leaves an orange-yellow colour in the liver years after the disease is supposedly cured. Chemotherapy clogs the whole auric field and specially the liver. Radiation therapy turns the structured layers of the auric field ragged and burnt. If these are not attended to by healing, the physical body will have a much more difficult time healing itself. Different diseases affect different chakras. AIDS can clog the base and root chakra, and sometimes the entire field depending on the progress of the disease. Torn chakras are connected with cancer, rendering the patient much more vulnerable to outside influences.

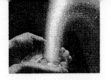

CHAPTER NINE

BUILDING AND STRENGTHENING THE CHAKRAS

Whereas exercises to strengthen the aura are about taking an overall look at our relationship to ourselves, chakra work is about the detail and is normally more technical. For example, the solar plexus chakra is often torn when a relationship ends in a disharmonious way. In a later chapter I discuss various case histories.

The overall view is that as we fulfil the law of life through purification of the threefold lower self and service to others, the centres are slowly and automatically unfolded and activated. By setting out deliberately to force the opening of the chakras, and to intensify their action through chanting and other so-called spiritual exercises designed to open us up, the subject may unleash energies which will tear and damage the physical tissues of the body, especially those of the nervous system and brain, thus leading to physical and emotional instability. The key that opens the centres lies quite simply in a steady orientation towards the soul, the divine nature of other people and a responsiveness to soul contact expressed through service.

CHAKRAS AND HEALING

Spiritual healing is possibly the most rewarding and challenging psychic ability. At its highest level, it can create peace and feelings of being in touch with the universe. Benefits can be felt immediately after beginning to learn it, but the skills continue to improve for years, as a constant challenge to keep growing. There are many forms of spiritual healing in existence, both from Western and Eastern philosophies. Chakra work and aura healing will be covered briefly here. Regardless of the form of healing used, the healer must put their own needs ahead of others' needs. A healer who only heals others whilst ceasing to care for their own welfare will burn out very quickly.

Healing others should not be used as a way of avoiding personal problems. While healing others can contribute to preparing to handle the self, it must not be done so totally that the healer tires and has a lower quality of life because of it. An exaggerated motive of self-sacrifice benefits no one in the long term. A healthy healer can do much more than an ill one.

Blocks in a certain chakra, either caused emotionally or by injury, often create problems in the related area of life. Cleaning the chakras out and re-energizing them helps overcome those problems. You cannot have a good composite structure – in other words a good aura – unless there is integrity in the individual chakras.

I would now like to discuss my work on clearing out chakras and to give practical examples. Through the chakras, the major nerve plexuses and the intricate network of fine nerves, we register those energies and forces which flow to us from a multitude of sources throughout the universe. At the same time, energies from the mental, emotional and etheric environment make their impress upon us, and as spiritual unfoldment proceeds we become increasingly sensitive to the prompting forces flowing to us expressed via our responsive free will.

Chakras both receive and transmit energies for creative or destructive purposes. A person working through an uncontrolled and highly developed solar plexus can create havoc in their environment. Another person working creatively through the throat or the heart chakras radiates peace and harmony in such a way that others are uplifted and quietly inspired by their presence.

CHAKRAS FROM THE PRACTITIONER'S POINT OF VIEW

This is a summary of my findings with regard to chakras. The aim is to have a balanced system. Openness in itself is not a virtue. It is of little value to have an open crown or third eye if the other chakras do not support them. There is just as much danger in spiritual over-ambitiousness as in spiritual torpor. Sometimes a chakra does not give a reading at all. This is when a person is not grounded. I call this the 'suspended' state. It often happens with the crown chakra when a person has given up one belief system and has not found something else to take its place.

Root (grounding)

Open. This belongs to a person who is ambitious. This ambition takes the form of a desire to succeed at their occupation. In its extreme form, such people are driven by their vision and have little time for relaxation. However, if combined with an open throat chakra and a balanced heart chakra the result can be a very productive life.

Balanced. I name this state the 'common sense' condition. The subject is realistic with regard to their aims and ambitions. They know they must earn a living. They enjoy their job but do not let it consume their lives. Their decisions are featured by common sense. They do not rush off and attempt a task which is unsuitable for them.

Closed. This happens when a person has given up. It is to be found in students who have not started their courses, in many unemployed people and those who have retired to a life of boredom. In this case, motivational counselling is vital.

Sacral (sexual)

Open. In our modern society very few sacral chakras are in a state of balance. Unfortunately, people do not have enough chances to create quality time for and with each other. Sex and intimacy cannot be rushed at the end of a hard day. An open chakra often occurs when an individual has torn away from a relationship. This is accompanied by phantasies and emotionally disturbing thoughts. Healing and reconciliation are necessary in this case.

Balanced. These occur in good stable relationships.

Closed. These occur when a person has withdrawn from the possibility of a relationship. They may have decided to become celibate, or to withdraw from relationships until the right situation comes along. This is the council of wisdom.

I have advised so many people to take time out and go for a walk in the country and get away from the pressures of big city existence. If the other chakras are not balanced it is very unlikely that there will be harmony in this chakra.

Solar Plexus

Open. This is the most telling chakra with regard to relationships. A sudden end of an affair or a marriage will inevitably tear at the chakra. This leaves a gaping wound and all forces – disharmonious or otherwise – can gain admittance. A person will feel down for no reason. They do not know who they are or what their purpose is. Then, as suddenly as it appears, the mood will disappear and they will be back to their normal self. In this case healing is required. This healing is the combined effect of understanding the situation and the interposition of the gifts of the healer. Unfortunately it is quite rare for the individual to have enough strength to make the changes and heal their own wounds.

Balanced. A person who knows how to enjoy a good relationship without being possessed or wishing to be possessive. Energy drainers are soon detected and dismissed. Balanced people have a capacity to enjoy a wide variety of social relationships.

Closed. A closed chakra is a sign that after a relationship, the person has withdrawn to avoid further punishment. They feel that something is leaking and so compensate by withdrawal. Here like the closed heart, they often miss out on social opportunities saying to themselves "that won't happen to me again". The problem is that they close off too well and if you close in a pain, it festers.

Heart

Open. So beautiful and so dangerous. It's not a question of if a person has been hurt in a relationship, but how. These people see the world as they want it to be. They ignore negative indications and try to the bitter end to make them work, even when the signs of rigour mortis are there. 90% of the open hearts that I find belong to women. This may be because of the desire to give the benefit of the doubt.

Balanced. A balanced heart is the power house of the aura. Able and willing to give to others and yet having energy to spare. Such people need to be encouraged to have time for themselves. Their fears of being selfish are always ungrounded. I often distinguish between being 'selfish' and 'self-regarding'. Selfish excludes other people's needs. Self-regard is necessary to preserve the balance between work and play and between the need for one's own space, and to share fellowship with others. A person who 'gives' all the time quickly becomes exhausted.

Closed. I called this the 'snail in the shell' situation. An individual who has been hurt will retreat within themselves to avoid further battering. The problem is that they miss out on normal social intercourse and may even turn down invitations to social gatherings. This action will be combined with a lack of self-esteem. Such people need to be gently led back into the mainstream of society and need to learn the value of laughter and play.

Throat

Open. The throat chakra is meant as a meeting and blending place for the awareness that is in the crown and those energies which flow up from the root. An open chakra is very rare, because so many people compromise their creativity for the sake of security or career. The open chakra is almost always a positive sign. The subject shows great enthusiasm for work. "There are not enough hours in the day" is the common complaint. It is common to find the impulse for service to the community to be instinctive with this chakra open.

Balanced. In these subjects the seeking for fulfilment through having an outlet for all one's particular abilities is acknowledged. These people need to be true to themselves. Here the talents 'come of age' and the subject is well on the path to a useful integration in society.

Closed. Invariably these people are searching either for a meaningful job or a creative outlet. They are frustrated and in need of a means of expression. Their present employment lacks long-term viability. They do not see their way ahead to a career of satisfaction. They need career guidance – a matter for a career analyst.

Third Eye

Open. Unless supported by other chakras, this can be very dangerous. I have found this with exercises to increase perception. The pineal gland is a powerful organ and should be respected. It is particularly important that its development is not forced. It will become more prominent when the aura can handle the mass of information that comes in. An immature or unstable person will pick up masses of information from other people, not necessarily of a desirable sort. It is much better for the third eye to lag behind other chakras (for example the heart) than to lead.

Balanced. The ideal condition. The subject is able to perceive qualities in others without the need for a verbal exchange. They can tell if others are lying or hiding material. I have known several teachers and people working in credit control departments of companies who have this chakra balanced. They inevitably know when students or customers are being deceptive.

Closed. More often than not, a closed chakra is due to lack of confidence rather than an intrinsic inability to use the intuition. Many married women whose husbands are not interested in the spiritual life have low esteem. They are not able to share their feelings. Their intuitive attempts are dismissed as merely their own imagination. No wonder their confidence is reduced. The pineal gland cannot function effectively under such circumstances.

Crown

Open. An open chakra is to be found only in a very small percentage of subjects. This correlates with high spiritual development, an almost sublime love of their fellow humans, and is seldom reached through the efforts of one lifetime.

Balanced. This shows an ability and desire to trust our creator for provision of the needs of life. Such people will always be provided for, provided they trust in their creator and maintain their integrity. They instinctively know what is right and have a well developed conscience.

Closed. The client has lost their way spiritually and has rejected God. Frequently, lapsed Roman Catholics are to be found in this category. In other cases, there is a desire to believe but it is not fanned by the enthusiasm and faith of other people. Belief cannot take place on a solitary basis, at least not until the individual has become strong.

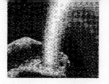

CHAPTER TEN

LIMITS AND DANGERS OF WORKING WITH THE AURAS AND CHAKRAS

What influences us to 'be' the way we are, and what has the power to constitute and assemble our aura? There is no avoiding the fact that, as St. Paul said, we are "members one of another". This deceptively homely analogy of the human body reveals the complex nature of our interconnectedness.

We can only become aware of our true self if we are free from psychic contamination. Often, my clients complain that they suddenly became depressed 'for no reason'. "I don't know what came over me", is the complaint. Some negative effects are due to an open or torn chakra, and in this case the chakra needs to be repaired and healed. In other cases, the whole aura is affected in general and this is where some form of psychic self-defence is required. We have all experienced being 'drained' by another person's presence in the room. We can feel the effect of jealousy, fear and hatred within our aura.

THE DANGERS INHERENT IN WORKING ON OURSELVES

Any type of ambition, including spiritual aspiration can be dangerous. Students talk of 'raising the kundalini' as if this were some sort of acquisition. Even to think of such aims takes preparation and spiritual refinement. Chakras need to be handled with care. Over-stimulation of any chakra activates the pranic forces of that chakra and can open doorways to other areas of consciousness. Once you have got the consciousness, what do you do with it?

'There is a time for everything, and for everything there is time'. Chakras develop in their own time when they are ready. As you would not try to precipitate the germination of seeds by putting them in an oven, so you would not try to force 'spiritual development' by exercises. When there is alignment between mind, body and spirit, the development will take place of its own accord in the sequence which will help us to enhance not only our own lives but the quality of life of others.

There could be nothing more damaging than suddenly becoming clairvoyant or suddenly obtaining the gift of healing. The ego is frail and the power gained would render the individual impossible to live with, or even ineffective in his or her daily life.

HOW CAN WE STRENGTHEN OUR ENERGY FIELD?

As we practise physical self-defence to protect the body, so we need psychic self-defence to protect the aura. There are many exercises that we can follow. Positive self-visualization is always good, as is the absence of negative thinking. We should also learn to be in the right places at the right time. Those of you that believe in spirit guides know that our welfare is their concern and if we listen to the small voice, we will be directed aright.

The power of positive visualisation cannot be over-estimated. We all know people who seem to draw bad luck to them. Well, the opposite is also possible. Here is an exercise that you can try a few times each day.

Stand erect and breathe deeply and evenly, relaxing from top to toe. Relax your whole body starting from the head working slowly down to the bottom of the feet. Visualize yourself being surrounded by an envelope of bright blue light that extends about nine inches from every point on the surface of your body. Whilst holding this image in your mind, visualize white light above your head. Imagine that this white light is becoming brighter and brighter.

Whilst this is in your mind, think of the highest standards of faith, morality and behaviour. Then feel the white light above you permeating your entire being like sparks from a firework. The outer shell of your aura should be blue light filled with white light. Concentrate on this image as long as you can. Become aware of sharply defined images. Finally close down, let the image fade slowly while believing that it is not fading from reality itself.

THE USE OF BREATHING

Very few of us know how to breathe. We 'take breaths', we pant, we gasp, but very few see breathing as a method of becoming one with the rhythms of the universe. Here is an exercise that anyone can do.

Wearing comfortable clothing and being free from anything that might disturb you, allow yourself to be. If you have problems on your mind, write them down on a piece of paper and lay them aside.

For the first five minutes generally relax. There is nothing more pointless than 'trying' to relax! Think about what you are going to do and look forward to it. Identifying what you believe in brings a certain guidance and protection. Believe that only good spirits are around, giving their love and protection to you. Uplift your spirit and envision your higher self.

Now try some controlled breathing. Begin the breathing with several large full breaths, all the way to the lower abdominal area. Then breathe in for a count of eight and then hold for a count of four. Exhale for a count of eight then hold for a count of four. Continue in this way, which you will find very relaxing and trance inducing. It also begins to bring you a regulated pattern of energy for the work ahead. Continue the breathing throughout the meditation. And don't worry if you forget it for a time. Just pick it up again and continue. The main thing is that you are comfortable with the method.

Beginning with the crown chakra, feel it opening up and becoming charged with light. Move to the third-eye chakra. Open and charge this. Do the same with the throat chakra. Continue with the other chakras. If there is resistance then stay with it, breathing in and out and focusing the incoming, good energy into that chakra. Try to balance the energy given to each chakra.

Turn your attention to the place of visions, the third eye. When the chakras are all open, and you are continuing to breathe as stated, it is time to look within. Find the place inside your mind where you see pictures, where you daydream. Hold a simple object such as an orange, or the sun, inside your mind. Do this for at least five minutes whilst you become quiet and just practice observing whatever may arise in this space. Do not give it any credence, and do not make any judgements. If you perceive any negative thoughts, just bless them. Do not endow them with power they do not need to have.

When you feel ready, spend a few moments closing down. Continue the breathing. Go back down the chakras, as before, diminishing the energy, dimming the light, so to speak, and envisioning that you are closing each spatial door as you do so. Then just quietly close the spiritual doors.

This meditation should be done with eyes closed but at the start a dim light can be on. It can be done in a group setting and is an excellent group meditation practice. Keep a quiet mind throughout.

These are just a sample of the exercises used to balance the chakras. There are many others but these are given for simplicity. Anyone can do them safely and alone.

For some people, such exercises are sufficient to bring about peace of mind. For others, however, personal intervention is more appropriate. Some choose the services of those in the mainstream of conventional therapy. Others choose alternative or complementary methods of support.

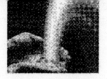

Chapter Eleven

Chakras in Everyday Life

Why is a sensitive consultation effective?

There are five stages of intervention which should guide any person seeking to assist another to strengthen their aura. These comprise a 'cascade' and careful use will prevent some of the frequently reported unpleasant and counter-productive side effects.

Minimalist stance. This relies on the client using the session to address the problem with minimal interference. It requires that the counsellor simply 'be', i.e., to listen. They can sit with the client and meditate, or listen to music or talk about everyday things. There is much anecdotal evidence for the success of this method. If we look back over our lives and remember the times that we have been helped, the person who helped us was not aware that they had been able to assist. Very often the feeling of freedom to share or express our concerns is sufficient to cause a breakthrough in our perception of our problem. One of our main burdens is not having the confidence or the perception to know when sharing a situation will have the most beneficial effect. The silent mixing of auras is often all that is necessary to ease the situation.

Observation stance. Making no value judgements the counsellor asks the client to expand and explain the situations. Here the counsellor listens to the client, commenting where appropriate.

There are three aspects of listening: what the person says; what they are asking; what they really need. What are the deep issues behind the questions? What is the client able to respond to or achieve? The counsellor keeps all this in mind and believes that the power of the observation will draw out and clarify the solution. The counsellor knows that the real validity lies in teasing out from the client lines of determination to make changes for themselves and take responsibility for their own actions.

Suggestion stance. The counsellor has done all the above but feels that not enough has been achieved. He may feel that the client needs more motivation so he will suggest various options of activity.

Directional stance. In the case of the client finding difficulty in making their own decision, or being unable to emerge from a self-destructive phase, the counsellor may direct them in a particular course. This is the least desirable and an approach of last resort. "Bearing in mind the circumstances, this would seem to be the only alternative". "Perhaps it would be wise to leave your boy-friend". "Seek a divorce". "See your solicitor". In a more extreme mode, this may take the guise of an order. The effect is the same. A hierarchy has been established, one of dependence on the counsellor, hopefully of a temporary nature.

The goal is to say the minimum as a counsellor and let the client achieve the most. Then it is their victory and more empowering for that.

WHAT IS A 'SENSITIVE READING?'

A sensitive interpretation involves not only our own psychology and training as practitioners, but the colours of the aura of the client and the information radiating from it. It also involves the influence of spiritual beings not in a body (discarnate entities), the Akashic records (an account of everything that has ever happened or been thought of) and cosmic consciousness, or an awareness of the relationship of homo sapiens on Planet Earth to the whole universe, not only the physical Universe, but the universe of thought.

WHAT IS THE 'UNIVERSE OF THOUGHT?'

We all need to inscribe meaning into the world and so we construct an edifice of sense. We may base this around convenience, comfort, security, the need for love. If this world view is adequate and true, then we will find peace of mind for us and for those we touch. If our world view is not adequate, then we will spread disharmony. Many of us construct an artificial universe based not on a vision of a better life but as a reaction against the hurts and fears of our immediate past experiences.

This is the way that the mind tries to dissociate from pain and separate itself from the surrounding circumstances. This breeds fear which in turn breeds aggression. This negative disposition has the power to affect not only our own energy body but our relationships with others. As many scientific papers have shown, due to the nature of telepathy, we are all linked. The 'universe of thought' is the sum total of all experiences of human beings on the planet. It's like a cocktail and to live and thrive in this is increasingly more difficult as the world situation deteriorates. Not only the individual but the world has an aura.

ARE INTUITIVE SKILLS RELEVANT TO SOLVING PROBLEMS?

Intuition provides an extra breadth and depth to the situation at hand. Working with chakras and auras involves, for most non-skilled people, the seeking of advice from others, and as such there is a degree of vulnerability. This is true for any type of consultation – be it a doctor, psychotherapist or priest.

Should we say to ourselves "I will not go to a psychic or sensitive because I may be misled"? This would not be an intelligent course of action because you may lose out on the opportunity to learn more about yourself. The answer as we have seen is to trust your own intuition so that it may guide you accurately.

HOW DO I ARRANGE A CONSULTATION?

The answer is to go along with an open state of mind. First, if you possibly can, go on the recommendation of someone who has been and received benefit. Ask them about the session – the length, the cost, and if you are allowed to ask questions. Is the session taped? When you make an appointment, confirm all these details. This will save embarrassment later.

HOW CAN I MAKE SURE A SENSITIVE COUNSELLING SESSION IS WORTHWHILE?

It may help you to focus your mind by writing down questions beforehand. In the excitement of the session it is easy to forget a vital point. Some sensitives will take telephone calls at future times but it is better to ask questions while their mind is fully focused on you. Do not be too ambitious about what can be done. Let the session have a life of its own. Very often the sensitive will tell you what you already know. This can be very helpful and confirming, giving you a new strength. Learn to allow new knowledge to become part of you in a dynamic way.

When readings are less than successful the most likely reason is that there is an unrealistic level of expectation on the part of the client. A sensitive may disturb your self-image. He or she cannot perform an act of healing on your behalf. They can enlighten, encourage, stimulate and inform but in the final analysis it is you that must do the work. Will you lose your independence by seeking a consultation? Why should you? Given time, we can all work out our problems. The reality is that we are in a world of time, and 'spare' time is what we do not have. A good sensitive reading will diminish the time needed to come to grips with something, and resolve it cleanly, enabling the client to do the necessary work.

The accuracy of readings works not only according to the ability of the sensitive but the 'merit' of the request. If, for example, a person has asked the same question many times of many sensitives, has been told the answer and refused to act on it, the inspiration of a sensitive will not function. The universe has given the answer – or a working answer, and it has been ignored. How can the universe give of itself again?

The mistake is to think of information coming directly from the brain of the sensitive. It comes via the mind – which is not a personal thing, though it lodges in the individual and can be used by those sensitive enough to receive, translate and transmit. The client, like the sensitive, needs an open mind.

WHAT IS AN 'OPEN MIND?'

This term has nothing to do with naivity. In another way, you could say "I will put all preconceived notions about my problem or situation to one side and I will not let them interfere with the material that comes out of this session". Honesty, and lack of defensiveness, is a vital part of the client's attitude.

Similarly, the sensitive must also have an open mind. Irrespective of the appearance of the client or anything they say, the sensitive must ignore all irrelevancies and simply 'tune in' to the life-force of the client, the dynamic interplay between the demands of daily life and the 'pull' of the soul.

IS IT WISE TO RECORD THE SESSION?

Some of us have very good memories and have no need for a mechanical aid. However, I have observed that the average person remembers about 30% of what they are told. When a point is made that is of emotional significance you tend to forget the next two or three points. Although you hear them they are not absorbed. A tape recorder is often a good idea but please try it out first. There is nothing more irritating than a client having borrowed a machine from a friend, fiddling around for five minutes trying to make it work!

WHAT DO I DO IF THERE IS A DISAGREEMENT?

The sensitive will see the problem from a different point of view to the client. When you are living within a situation you are so absorbed with the detail that you do not see, or may not want to see, the pattern or trend. If there is a difference of opinion, the client should ask the counsellor to repeat or explain the idea using other words. If the difference still persists, it may be due to fundamental misunderstandings of language, and this should be discussed immediately. Very often, a disagreement is part of the process of healing. You as the client do yourself no service if you disagree with a point without saying so. Never be afraid to speak out and take an active part in the session.

WHAT DO I DO IF I DO NOT UNDERSTAND WHAT IS BEING SAID?

Communication is a subtle art. Two people can hear the same statement and interpret it in a different way. This is because their life experiences are different. A good example is the word 'sex' or the word 'God'. Every word has an emotional element attached to it. The client should ask the sensitive to repeat what was said. No offence will be taken. A professional who loves their subject will want it to be communicated to others and they will repeat, using other words and phrases, until you understand their point. You are paying for the session. It is your right to understand what is being said. If a tape recording has been made, make a note to play it through after the session. The chances are that you were so occupied with one point that you will have missed another.

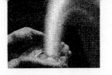

CHAPTER TWELVE

AURAS AND CHAKRAS FROM A SPIRITUAL VIEWPOINT

One of the traps that we can easily fall into is spiritual pride. If I say to you "I am spiritual" then I am probably not. This is hubris – spiritual pride – talking. A genuinely spiritual person would not be able to say that. There is no point in developing our spiritual life – or strengthening our aura – just for the sake of it. There not only has to be a goal, but a vision of us as we are designed to be. Let's see what it is – and what it is not.

We have learned something of the need for spiritual integrity. This word means wholeness, soundness, uprightness, honesty and is related to the word 'integrate' – to be a complete whole by the combination of parts. Imagine four photographic negatives of the same person. If laid one over the other, they would seem as one. If one photograph is out of shape then the whole is unclear. It is the same with our bodies.

If our physical, mental, spiritual and emotional bodies 'fit' on each other then we become integrated automatically. In order for us to do so we need to be aware – or conscious – of the functioning of our various parts and their relationships to each other. Accordingly, 'high' consciousness is a simultaneous awareness of our many different and contrasting aspects. In technical language, we cannot have 'monopolar' consciousness. That is why we cannot neglect any aspect of ourselves nor should we avoid facing any pain, since that provides the very clues which will culminate in spiritual progress.

Different people look at life in different ways; we all have our own interpretation of the things we experience. The classic example is how some people see the cup as half full, while others see it as half empty. How we interpret our reality brings a certain quality, or lack of it, to our lives. When we truly heal a physically or emotionally painful event in our lives, our interpretation of the event changes, and we increase our potential to enjoy life and participate in it.

We have habitual patterns for how we interpret events, some of which may be limiting us and causing us further pain. If we can bring these patterns to consciousness, we can see them more clearly and then be in a position to make choices about whether to follow the same pattern, or begin to lay the foundation for a new one.

Any event that we experience travels through our energy body via our chakra system. You will recall that the energy body is a field of energy that penetrates and surrounds the physical body, and this energy field contains the templates for our physical body, emotions, thoughts and spirituality. Located at specific points in this energy field are vortexes of energy called chakras as has been previously explained.

So, for example, not only does your second chakra nourish the physical body in the abdominal and lower back area, it also holds specific thought forms, belief systems and emotional energy, which have input into how you interpret what happens in your life. The energy of an event enters the first chakra where it is recorded as a physical fact. The energy from the event then moves through the chakra system, with each major chakra colouring the interpretation of the event in a certain way. If all our chakras are healthy, and not distorted or blocked in any way, the statement of fact will move through the system without impediment and the fact will become enlightenment when it gets to the seventh chakra.

The trouble is that our chakra system is usually not without some impediment somewhere. We begin to distort our energy fields and thus our chakras, early in life, as a reaction to what we perceive as painful events in childhood. Our goal as adults is to recognize these distortions, which become our defenses, and change them to more healthy ways of being. With conscious intention, we can do this; understanding how information travels through our chakra system is helpful to fulfil this task.

I'd like to give an example from everyday life to further illustrate the workings of the chakra and aura system.

Imagine that whilst buying a train ticket, you spill your money over the floor. The person behind complains bitterly that you are holding him up and that he has a train to catch. When you fumble with picking up the money he abuses you in front of others and pushes his way in front of you.

Everything that happens in our vicinity affects us. The only question is 'how'. On a good day, you may be able to shrug this off and say, he's having a bad day, which means that what happened got through your first three chakras without a hitch. However, there's more to the process than that, and there's also the fact that you may not be able to detach from what happened so easily; you may have a defensive reaction yourself to the event that occurred.

We'll take this event through the chakras step by step. In the first (base) chakra, what happens is recorded as a physical fact. In a clear first chakra, this would simply be the statement of what happened, as described above, as though an impartial observer reported the event. However, a distorted interpretation would define the event from a limited viewpoint. For example, not feeling safe. You might say: that man verbally abused me. I didn't do anything wrong. He is mean and nasty – in effect, the enemy. Now there are two sides, set for a battle, 'the me vs. them'. Consciousness begins colouring the event immediately, interpreting it as one of someone being abusive, defining a perpetrator and a victim. This statement that comes out of the first chakra is not at all that of the impartial observer, in fact quite the opposite.

Depending on your habitual defensive reactions, you may now want to run and hide, cry, whine and blame or go after the guy and teach him a lesson. This plays into how the second chakra is interpreting the event. The second chakra computer is programmed to deal with what we perceive as power issues. Who has more? You or the man in the street? The poor-me victim consciousness will say: "The complainer is a bad guy. If only he hadn't done that, I would feel better. If only this were not happening". A more aggressive interpretation would be to decide that the abuser has to be taught a lesson, and you're just the one to do it. You'll show him who has more power, even if it's just in talking about the situation, and proving to others how bad he was. Of course, there are many reactions between these two extremes; but in each case, you are not feeling too good about the event. You are still hooked into it, it is having a lot of authority in your life at the moment and it is disturbing your day.

However, if your second chakra is undistorted, you interpret the event in a detached manner. A healthy second chakra sees a power struggle as an illusion and brings you the understanding that all people are in your life for a reason, no matter the packaging they come in. You may not know or understand why this event occurred, but you understand that everyone you run across has something to do with your growth. So you leave behind the notion that someone in this scenario has to have more power than the other, and you might decide that that was not a pleasant experience, but that lessons can be learned from it. "That man came into my life so I could grow, and I can honour him for his participation in my growth process." Now you don't need your battle gear, you are not hooked into the man's behaviour and the effect it had and the event does not have the ability to affect the remainder of your day. Honouring the complainer in this way does not mean that you condone his aggressive behaviour. It simply means that you know there is more to this story than meets the eye, and he is part of a message the universe is trying to send you. You become curious about the event, and his behaviour, rather than reacting to it as a victim.

If your self-esteem is healthy, your third – solar plexus – chakra will be also, and you will continue to interpret the event in this way and think "I am worthy of respect and dignity from myself and everyone else. I will not take on as truth any-thing the man said about me. I know I am okay. I can choose to set boundaries for myself so that I do not have to be around people who do not respect me. Had the man continued to behave in the way he was behaving, I could have removed myself from his presence if I needed to".

Your healthy sense of yourself allows you to know that you are okay, not bad, that your worth is not dependent on what someone else says and you know that you can take care of yourself. Compare this to what comes out of a distorted third chakra. "Who should have protected me? What if the things he said are true? Why didn't he like me? What's wrong with me? I feel terrible." These distorted third chakra statements may or may not be conscious. You may merely be aware that you are angry and/or hurt, and feeling awful, and not be aware of the fact that you are allowing your self-worth to be called into question by the remarks of a stranger.

Now we come to the fourth chakra, the energy centre of the heart. The heart chakra is healthy when we can love and forgive, both ourselves and others. A healthy heart chakra would report on the event in this way: "I know that the complainant's behaviour comes from a place of his own pain, and that both he and I were merely actors in a little drama. That man must have been suffering in some way, because it is our pain that makes us not respect the dignity of others. I can open my heart to him, have compassion for him, even though I have no idea what his pain is about. I can forgive him for his actions, and in doing so, I clear myself of his negative energy. I am free." This chakra, the heart, is a crucial one. If we let the energy of the event flow through the heart fully by being compassionate and forgiving, the energy can move into the upper chakras, which further defines for us how we can learn and grow from what happened. If we close the heart and stop any further progress, the energy of the event repeatedly circles in a negative way through the first three chakras. How easy is it for us to forgive? How easy to detach from painful events and be compassionate so that we can let them go? This piece usually does not come naturally, and we need to have a conscious intention to open fully to our loving and forgiving energy. If we can, the event automatically transforms and the energy of it moves into the upper chakras where we can extract more of its gifts to continue our evolutionary process.

If we close our hearts, we say things like: "I will never forgive. He doesn't deserve forgiveness. He ruined my day, my ability to be happy. I certainly could never love that man." Unfortunately, the closed heart statements are many times more familiar to us.

In almost every spiritual belief system, great emphasis is placed on the heart and the power of love, with the view set forth that we are here on this planet mainly to learn how to love and transform our experiences with the power of our love. I am sure everyone knows a story about the transformational power of loving and forgiving. The acts of loving ourselves and others, and forgiving ourselves and others have the most profound effects upon our life –- our physical health, our emotional and mental state, and our spirituality. The heart is indeed a crucible, an instrument of conversion, capable of evincing a compassion for the human condition, metabolizing the energy that moves through it into a new and higher frequency. This higher frequency energy equates with a higher consciousness. This is why the heart chakra is called the bridge between the lower three chakras, whose energies are concerned with how to live in the world of matter, and the upper three chakras, whose energies have a higher vibration and deal with the world of spirit.

If the heart chakra is closed, the energy of an event continuously recycles itself through our lower three chakras. We sometimes begin to relish the negative energy generated by an event. It may bring us power over people, sympathy, or allow us to continuously discharge anger in various inappropriate ways. With the heart closed, we can't access our forgiving energy, and we make a choice, consciously or unconsciously, to refuse to let go of the event. Consequently, there is no resolution; the experience remains in our energy fields, and in our lives, as unfinished business. The energies of our lower three chakras are re-routed into the negative belief systems triggered by the event. Sending our energy into negative belief systems takes it away from our healthy physical body, healthy emotional and mental state, and healthy spirituality. When we say "I can't forgive", ultimately, we end up paying for it with our cell tissue, as well as our peace of mind.

The open heart chakra, however, has a purifying effect on the energy moving through it, and that energy is then available to move into the upper three chakras. The fifth, or throat chakra, always brings us to an increased awareness of ourselves. The fifth chakra demands that we speak the truth, and part of that truth-speaking is an acknowledgment of our own issues, negative behaviours, and masks to the outer world. Also contained in the throat chakra is the energy of our will. Using our example of the ticket office incident, a healthy fifth chakra would relay to us a statement like: "I acknowledge how this incident tempts me to fall into my victim role. I have an addiction to playing the victim, and the victim energy that I carry attracts people like the complainer, who are addicted to playing perpetrator. However, I have the ability to stop myself from playing victim, and I refuse to allow myself to play victim right now. I refuse to buy into the belief that I am the 'good' victim, and that man is the 'bad' perpetrator."

Sometimes the concept that our passive victim energy can attract an aggressive perpetrator energy is difficult to accept. However, energetically, the perpetrator energy pattern and the victim energy pattern fit together like pieces of a puzzle, and on an unconscious level, these two patterns seek each other out. Without the transformative energies of the heart chakra, it is extremely difficult to admit that our victim role played just as big a part in the incident as did the perpetrator. Victim and perpetrator are merely two poles on the same continuum; we all have both energies in us, but probably act out one more strongly than the other. In looking at ourselves honestly (using the energies of the throat chakra in a healthy way), it is our responsibility to acknowledge our inappropriate patterns and behaviours. The forgiving energy of the heart chakra allows us to do this without self-judgment, and use our will to get on with cleaning up our act. The fact that we have negative, reactionary behaviours does not mean we are bad! It simply means that we are human. What is important is what we do about the behaviour once we have noticed and acknowledged it.

Compare this concept with statements from the distorted throat chakra. "I want justice! This was not my fault! I am completely innocent and none of my energy was involved in this incident. I didn't do anything wrong; the complainer was wrong!" These statements merely push the energy of the incident back down into the second chakra, which will take care of the retribution that the person is demanding. When we do not learn from an event, the Universe simply gives us more of a similar kind of incident, until we finally do learn something.

When the throat chakra 'speaks the truth', the sixth chakra, also called the third eye, begins to 'see the truth'. On a physical level, the sixth chakra regulates the organs of sight, the eyes; it also has to do with insight, and seeing events symbolically, not just in a literal way. The interpretation of events symbolically allows us to understand them on a deeper level, a more conscious level. In a way that has little to do with the linear mind, we begin to understand events from an expanded perspective. It is as if we can step outside our lives, and see that the experiences that come to us are exactly what we need for our growth. We find meaning and insights in our lives. Our job here is to see the situation so clearly, that we empower ourselves and are able, simply by our presence, to comfort and uplift others so that they can then empower themselves.

So the healthy sixth chakra makes statements like these in the station incident. "One of my life tasks is to learn to give up the victim energy. I accept this in my life. That's why I needed to experience the complainant shouting at me – to practice not playing victim! I know that I can use this situation to empower myself, and I know that in doing so, I give others the opportunity to empower themselves." Meanwhile, the distorted sixth chakra whines: "why does this keep happening to me? My life is always like this".

When energy cannot move freely through the seventh, or crown, chakra, the statement that emerges is a simple one: "life is not fair". You hear children say this all the time, which is understandable, because up until adolescence they usually are developing their three lower chakras. Energetically, they don't have the 'equipment' of the developed seventh chakra to truly understand the meaning of life, and reject the notion that 'life is not fair'. As adults, we do have the energies of our seventh chakra available to us if we wish to use them. When our crown chakra is open, we know, without proof or explanation, that there is a Divine plan, and we are part of it. We are able to accept life's experiences, even when they are very painful or make absolutely no sense from the perspective human linear mind. It is the energies of this chakra that help us get through trauma and crisis, through the dark nights of the soul, without breaking. Here we come to terms with the tragedy of the human condition, and are still able to find joy and peace in our lives.

If the energy of the difficult incident travels through our chakra system unimpeded, by the time it gets to the seventh chakra, the statement is: "I trust in the Divine plan of the Universe. I know that I have been given a gift in the form of the incident in the ticket office, and I know that I have grown from it. I am better for what happened. We are all One. We're back to the first chakra again: all Is One. The incident is finished; it was simply another lesson in Life's classroom". Rather than have some amount of our energy tied up somewhere with this incident, we now have that same amount of energy available for enjoying life, for pleasure. The choice is ours.

WHAT IS WHOLENESS OR TRANSCENDENCE?

So long as the life-force circulates through the left and right channels the human body, mind and spirit is moved forward through the ordinary ebb and flow of consciousness. However, mind and time stand still when the life current enters the axial channel, and there is only the bliss of reality. Both the mind and life-force are mingled like milk and water. Where the life force is active, there is mental activity. When one is stilled, the other is stilled as well. When one or both are active, a host of senses are active. When both are quiescent, the state of liberation is attained.

HOW DO WE VERIFY PSYCHIC OR PARANORMAL PHENOMENA?

Among scientists, auras are most definitely included in the list of banned topics. They say that seeing the aura is actually an after-effect of staring, more to do with auto-suggestion, coupled with the over-stimulation of the rods and cones, than any other reason. Therefore, they say, people who claim to see them are deluding themselves. To address this matter in a positive manner involves ridding one's mind of negative emotions. "The oldest emotion known to man is fear, and the strongest emotion is fear of the unknown". This applies particularly to psychic phenomena.

The conventional scientific stance can be summed up as follows:

1. I do not understand this class of phenomenon. 2. If I were to understand it, I would have to shift my paradigms. 3. If I did, my colleagues would perhaps laugh at me, and my grant applications would be threatened. 4. I will close my eyes to anything that does not fit in with my perception of the universe. 5. People who do seek understanding through religion or psi are inadequate in some way.

Note the objective and rational descriptions! When I hear this I wonder what they are afraid of. There is a danger in global rubbishing of a phenomena such as healing or clairvoyance. If you rubbish a subject you also by implication rubbish its history. Mocking healing is therefore to mock the work of Jesus Christ; mocking clairvoyance is to mock the work of Edgar Cayce, an American who gave thousands of diagnosis – often using strange medicines – which worked when conventional medical prescriptions had failed. That's a laser beam which is likely to turn into a boomerang for these detractors.

Those who hope for a rational pragmatic response from so-called investigators should look carefully. Many 'investigators' are in fact debunkers who have made up their mind that all psychics are frauds and that the only world of reality is the conventional world of science, where the mind is bound by and contained within the physical body. Any evidence which purports to show to the contrary is ignored or dismissed. The conclusion is quite clear. They will hang on to their old paradigms like a dog to a bone. If the world is greater than they allow themselves to think, then could they manage the change?

I do have some sympathy with this. When I first realized that rather than the mind being contained in the body, the body was simply the (relatively) solid part in the middle of the mind, it took me literally years to adapt to this and its implications. After 20 years I still catch myself thinking in the 'old' way, and that's with working full time in the psychic field. What chance does the conventional scientist have, let alone the one who has to seek grants from his or her rather conservative peer group? It is interesting how many scientists and researchers suddenly develop an interest in psychic material after they retire.

Parapsychological investigation and scientific investigation should follow the same rules and agreement on this must take place between the various camps before meaningful dialogue can take place. The rules of observing, recording, correlating and deducing should be well noted. You cannot jump steps in your enthusiasm and hope that no one will notice.

However, all is not lost. It is worth dwelling on the nature of a possible relationship between the traditional scientist and the parapsychologist of which the research into auras is a part.

Parapsychological and paraphysical matters are those in which an immense number and types of people are taking an interest. Parapsychology is interesting mainly because of the possible implications. To list a few examples, psi phenomena suggest (a) that what science knows about the nature of the universe is incomplete; (b) that the presumed capabilities and limitations of human potential have been underestimated; (c) that fundamental assumptions and philosophical beliefs about the separation of mind and body may be incorrect; and (d) that religious assumptions about the divine nature of 'miracles' may have been mistaken.

Some researchers regard the current findings of parapsychology as having a wide variety of important implications, including implications about the spiritual nature of humankind. This applies in their minds even if the supporting data is not there.

In general, physicists tend to be interested in parapsychology because of the implication that we have an inadequate understanding about the nature of space and time and the transmission of energy and information. Biologists are interested because psi implies the existence of additional, unexplained methods of sensing the world. Psychologists are interested for what psi implies about the nature of perception and memory. Philosophers are interested because psi phenomena specifically address many age-old philosophical problems, including the role of the mind in the physical world, and the nature of the objective vs. the subjective.

Theologians and the general public tend to be interested because personal psi experiences are often accompanied by feelings of profound, ineffable meaning. As a result, psi is thought by some to have spiritual implications.

From the materialistic perspective, which is one of the foundations of the scientific world view, human consciousness is nothing but an emergent product of the functioning of Brain, Body, and Nervous System (BBNS). That is, no matter how different mind may seem from solid stuff like bodies, it is generated solely by the electrochemical functioning of the BBNS, and so it is absolutely dependent on it. When the BBNS dies, so does consciousness. From this perspective, claims of survival of bodily death, or ghosts, or apparitions, must be due to wishful thinking. Furthermore, the limits of material functioning automatically determine the ultimate limits of mental functioning, thus ESP and PK appear to be impossible, given our current understanding about how the world works.

And yet, psi phenomena have occurred in all cultures throughout history. They continue to occur, and some of the reported phenomena have been persuasively verified using scientific methods. Because psi seems to transcend the assumed limits of material functioning, and therefore the BBNS, some interpret psi as supporting the idea that there is something more to mind than just the BBNS, that there is some sort of 'soul'.

This 'non-physical' aspect, an aspect that does not seem to be as tightly bounded by space or time as present scientific models require, might survive bodily death. If so, there may be important truths contained in some spiritual ideas and practices. Of course, parapsychology is a very long way from being able to say that a particular group are right about one thing or wrong about another.

There is a big difference between simply noting that the findings of parapsychology may have implications for spiritual concepts, versus the idea that parapsychologists are driven by some hidden spiritual agenda. Some critics of parapsychology seem to believe that all parapsychologists have hidden religious motives, and that they are really out to prove the existence of the soul. This is no more true than claiming that all chemists really harbour secret ambitions about alchemy, and thus their real agenda is to transmute base metals into gold. The reasons why serious investigators are drawn to any discipline are as diverse as their backgrounds.

WHY IS PARAPSYCHOLOGY SPECIAL?

What makes parapsychology special is the need to pay very close attention to 'conventional' explanations. This is because we've defined psi phenomena as exchanges of information that do not involve currently known (i.e., conventional) processes. For instance, we talk about "ESP" when people know about things going on in their environment without getting the information by seeing, hearing, touching, smelling, or through any other known sensory input, or without being able to figure out the 'target' information. We talk about PK when physical systems appear to react to people's intentions and there's no known physical contact between the person and the target.

Therefore, an important part of parapsychological research is eliminating known contact methods from laboratory setups and thinking carefully about them when evaluating reports of people's experiences. In ESP research, this requires knowing about the psychology of sensation, perception, memory, thinking, and communication, and about the biology and physics of sensation and movement. In PK studies, it is important to know about the physical characteristics of the target; how it works, and what might affect it. In field studies, and in most laboratory studies, it's important to know about the ways in which people can interact with each other. Of course, in field studies it is much more difficult to eliminate conventional explanations than it is in the laboratory because you can't set things up beforehand to eliminate conventional contact between the people and the targets.

Even when known contact methods are well controlled or eliminated, there is always the possibility that what we observe could have occurred by chance. That is, a person's apparent ESP knowledge about some distant event might be a random guess that just happens to resemble the target. Or, what looks like a PK effect on a physical system might be a random change in that system that just happens to occur at the right time. So it's important to know the statistical methods used to measure how likely it is that the event could have occurred by chance, and how to decide when that's so unlikely that it makes more sense to think there really was some kind of psi contact.

Sometimes field research is not concerned with whether the experiences people report were really psi phenomena, but instead asks questions like, "what do people report about experiences they think were psi; how does having these experiences affect their lives?; do people's psychological or cultural characteristics influence how likely they are to interpret experiences as psi?" This is straightforward anthropological, sociological, or psychological research and does not require the same kind of strict attention to eliminating conventional explanations.

The value of field research methods is that they investigate the experiences that people actually report. These include experiences such as precognitive dreams, out-of-body experiences, telepathic impressions, auras, memories of previous lives, hauntings and poltergeists and apparitions. Research on these issues results in information about incidence, phenomenology, demographic and psychological correlation of the experiences.

While field or spontaneous case research is less technical, and often more exciting to read, it is wise to avoid jumping to conclusions about the nature of psi from individual cases.

Such studies examine how people report or think about their experiences, not what those experiences actually are. However, because spontaneous case studies concentrate on the raw experience; they offer a valuable view of psi that is often missing in controlled laboratory experiments. Case studies provide a chance to discover the personal meanings and the psychodynamics underlying the experiences, which in turn may provide important hints as to possible mechanisms of psi.

An important goal of laboratory research is to determine the degree to which experiences reported in field and spontaneous-case research can be verified using current scientific methods. If they prove to be verifiable in the lab, the major intent of the lab work usually shifts from proof-oriented research to process-oriented; in which the goal is to discover the psychological, physiological, and physical mechanisms of each phenomenon.

WHAT ARE COMMON CRITICISMS OF RESEARCH INTO AURAS AND PARAPSYCHOLOGICAL PHENOMENA?

Constructive criticism is essential in science and is welcomed by the majority of active psi researchers. Strong scepticism is expected, and many parapsychologists are far more sceptical about psi than most outside scientists realize. However, it is not generally appreciated that some of the more vocal criticisms about psi are actually pseudo-criticisms.

It is commonly supposed by non-scientists that sceptical debates over the merits of psi research follow the standards of scholarly discussions. Unfortunately, this is not always the case. Disparaging rhetoric and ad hominem attacks arise too often in debates about psi. The science of parapsychology, and the way that science treats anomalies in general, is a fascinating topic that starkly illuminates the very human side of how science really works.

CRITICISM 1 Apparently successful experimental results are actually due to sloppy procedures, poorly trained researchers, methodological flaws, selective reporting, and statistics problems. There is therefore not a shred of scientific evidence for psi phenomena.

Response: these issues have been addressed in detail by analytic reviews of the experimental literature. The results unambiguously demonstrate that successful experiments cannot be explained away by these criticisms. In fact, research by Harvard University specialists in scientific methods showed that the best experimental psi research today is not only conducted according to proper scientific standards, but usually adheres to more rigorous protocols than are found in contemporary research in both the social and physical sciences. In addition, over the years there have been a number of very effective rebuttals of criticisms of individual studies, and within the past decade, experimental procedures have been developed that address virtually all methodological criticisms, even the possibility of fraud and collusion, by including sceptics in the experimental procedures.

CRITICISM 2 Psi phenomena violate basic limiting principles of science, and are therefore impossible.

Response: twenty years ago, this criticism was a fairly common retort to claims of psi phenomena. Today, with advancements in many scientific disciplines, the scientific world view is rapidly changing, and the basic limiting principles are constantly being redefined. In addition, the substantial empirical database in parapsychology now presents anomalies that simply won't go away; thus this criticism is no longer persuasive and is slowly disappearing. Given the rate of change in science today, assigning psi to the realm of the impossible now seems imprudent at best, foolish at worst.

CRITICISM 3 Parapsychology does not have a repeatable experiment.

Response: when many people talk about a repeatable psi experiment, they usually have in mind an experiment like those conducted in elementary physics classes to demonstrate the acceleration of gravity, or simple chemical reactions. In such experiments, where there are relatively few, well-known and well-controllable variables, the experiments can be performed by practically anyone, anytime, and they will work. But insisting on this level of repeatability is inappropriate for parapsychology, or for that matter, for most social or behavioral science experiments. Psi experiments usually involve many variables, some of which are poorly understood and difficult or impossible to directly control. Under these circumstances, scientists use statistical arguments to demonstrate repeatability; instead of the common, but restrictive view that if it's real, I should be able to do it whenever I want.

Under the assumption that there is no such thing as psi, we would expect that about 5% of well conducted psi experiments would be declared successful; (i.e., statistically significant) by pure chance. But suppose that in a series of 100 actual psi experiments we consistently observed that 20 were successful. This is extremely unlikely to occur by chance, suggesting that psi was present in some of those studies. However, it also means that in any particular experiment, there is an 80% probability of failure. Thus, if a critic set out to repeat a psi experiment to see if the phenomenon was 'real' and the experiment failed, it would obviously be incorrect to claim on the basis of that single experiment that psi is not real because it is not repeatable.

A widely accepted method of assessing repeatability in experiments is called meta-analysis. This quantitative technique is heavily used in the social, behavioural and medical sciences to integrate research results of numerous independent experiments. Starting around 1985, meta-analyses have been conducted on numerous types of psi experiments. In many of these analyses, results indicate that the outcomes were not due to chance, or methodological flaws, or selective reporting practices, or any other plausible normal explanations. What remains is psi, and in several experimental realms, it has clearly been replicated by independent investigators.

WHAT IS UNIQUE ABOUT THE HUMAN AURA?

"Man has no body distinct from his soul ..." William Blake.

The human aura occupies such a special place in psychic phenomena because we live partly in the physical world and partly in the spiritual world. Our human energy fields form a gateway between the two or, to put it another way, we are designed to straddle two types of reality – the temporal time-based reality and the spiritual eternal reality. To neglect the physical will bring about mental illness just as surely as neglecting the spiritual will bring about disorientation.

The spiritual world is beyond space, a grand statement with consequences. So far, few scientists have grasped all the implications including the great intellects such as Einstein, Neils Bohr and Stephen Hawking. The ideas are so rich that it would take a lifetime to simply realize their extent. For example in the spirit world, distance does not matter because there is no distance, so you cannot 'go' from A to B. Also, time does not exist so something does not happen before something else. A spiritual person lives not in time but in space and his or her focus is outside the realm of the intellect, and reminds us of the words in the Christian prayer book "The Peace of God, which passes all understanding".

Peace of mind is obtained by a marriage between the eternal world of the spirit and the soul, and the temporal world of physical matter. Both have an equally important part to play in our evolution. Neither should be dismissed in favour of the other in the same way that a vessel is not less important than the liquid it contains.

The difference in laws – and yet their complimentary nature – governing the two worlds should be understood. In the material world where laws of physics apply, a positive pole is always attracted to the negative one, and vice versa. Two positive poles repulse as do two negative poles.

The debate between matter and spirit will go on so long as man remains capable of thought. There is really no scientific or other method by which man can steer safely between the opposite dangers of believing too little or believing too much. To face such dangers is apparently our duty and to hit the right channel between them is the measure of our wisdom. People often conduct studies and throw away the data if it does not agree with their theory; the true scientist will throw away the theory! In such emotive fields, the predominance of rationality cannot be taken for granted.

In the spiritual world like is attracted to like. The positive pole attracts the positive one and so on. This should broaden our understanding of the human being. We can assume that there are three bases.

The first basis, the human body, belongs to the material world. It is mortal and subject to gradual decay and death. Yet no one would be alive without the second basis, the spiritual base, the moving spirit or the animating principle. The spirit – the spark of life – inspires the body from the moment it is born but the spirit alone, belonging as it does to a different world from the body, cannot 'co-exist' without a uniting basis. This is the third basis of the soul – that which harmoniously unites the spirit and the body and belongs to neither world.

This is the unique essence of the human soul revered and acknowledged in various philosophical and poetical works. The human soul belongs neither to the spiritual base nor to the material one. It is a self-sufficient substance. It is a translation, a gateway, a medium between one world and another. That is why it is – and has to be – eternal and immortal.

Underneath we all acknowledge the importance of this intrinsic part of our inner self. We talk of a 'good soul', a 'twin soul', he 'sold his soul', she put her 'heart and soul into her work' and so on.

A person's spirit is always with them, interpenetrating their body and in contrast to the above shows absolutely no reaction to emotional changes. Rather it depends on the psychological features the individual possesses. We talk of 'being out of spirits' or 'breaking someone's spirit'. It is interesting how the descriptions of the soul and spirit coincide with those of the inner and outer auras.

Our thoughts have power. Human ideas, words and emotions belong to the spiritual world. They possess form, direction and energy. We create millions of spiritual impulses each day. Most of them die, but some come to fruition. If we assume that thoughts are everywhere and fully realize the implications of this, we would be much more careful about the nature and harmony of our thinking. Thoughts are living things. They 'live' just a much as a cell, or a blade of grass. Thoughts do not live in time and space but are everywhere. This is why privacy is the supreme illusion. Nothing can really be hidden, though our mind may wish to think it so.

It behoves all thinking people to consider the role of the phenomenon of resonance, renamed by Rupert Sheldrake as 'morphic resonance'. The idea that there is the equivalent of critical mass in the realm of human experience is intriguing and lends weight to Jung's idea of the collective unconscious. Psychologists and scientists are finding considerable evidence in favour of the 'hundredth monkey' theory being applicable to humans as well as to animals. The original observation was that one monkey on an island learned to wash potatoes before eating them and then teaches others. As soon as one hundred monkeys wash potatoes, a certain critical limit of awareness is reached and monkeys on neighbouring islands will wash them without having gone through the conscious learning process. Thus this information travels without recourse to the normal channels of communication and does not depend on distance. Unlike normal radiations such as heat, this phenomenon does not obey the inverse square law. In simple terms the law states that if you move twice the distance from a radiating object, the power does not go down by half but by a quarter.

We may find that the aura works within a set of laws with which conventional science is only now beginning to grasp. The aura is an expression of the free will of humankind. It is the medium which connects our human field with the world around. Chakras are parts of the aura. They interconnect through the spine and act forwards and backwards through a series of cone movements. The integrity of the mind-body-spirit-soul combination determines the shape and form of the chakras, which in their turn determine the integrity of the aura.

Our aura can function on our behalf in a magnificent way. It can draw all the things to us for our good, or for our harm. It is quite literally our passport to life. Lack of understanding on an intellectual level should not preclude us from accepting as a working hypothesis that there is more to life than the physical. Physicality is but one mode. To exclude the others is to lead a very lonely and empty life.

And yet the ultimate stance is not one of the intellect. For those that believe, no explanation is necessary. For those that don't believe, no explanation is possible.

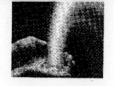

PART THREE

HOW TO READ THE AURA

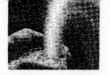

CHAPTER THIRTEEN

MY METHOD DESCRIBED

HOW TO READ THE AURA

I have developed this method of reading, over the years. Whilst it was growing, I did not recognize it as a distinct method but a bundle of experiences which seemed to fit. I have demonstrated this method with equal success in India, South Africa, Finland, Ireland and the UK – an interesting pointer to the universality of the human character.

The method is based on the following elements:

1. The radiations of a cocktail of fields – some of which are bioenergetic in nature – from any living thing.
2. The fact that these fields do not appear to obey the inverse square law. This means that they do not get more weak and chaotic the further the detector is from the source. All that is required is a mind able to focus strongly.
3. The ability of our central nervous system to detect 'atmospheres' around us.
4. The observation that the aura or subtle environment is particularly differentiated around the hands.
5. The further observation that the aura, influenced as it is by thought, 'knows' what its main needs are in order to develop itself. We have all had the experience of a 'needy person' pulling at us. This is not an intellectual process!

INITIAL MEASUREMENT WITH THE VOLTMETER

This is a most useful and telling indication as to the type of client that the practitioner is to be faced with in the interview. We speak of someone being left-brain dominant or right-brain dominant.

Left brainness represents the logical, sequential, materially orientated part of the brain in contrast to the right brain, focused as it is on intuition, imagination, feeling, emotions and humour.

Ideally, both hemispheres of a human subject will function equally effectively. That is the function of mediation. What may we learn from the animal kingdom in this respect? Interestingly a Russian research group led by L.M. Mukhametov discovered through electroencephalograms that in the case of bottle-nosed dolphins, hemispheres sleep one at a time. One of their animals spends 42.4% of his day alternating sleep between the hemispheres and only 0.8% of the time with both hemispheres asleep at once. While we can be certain that human brain hemispheres would never exhibit such gross difference in activity, the evidence that one mammalian brain can so readily switch dominance suggests that humans may also shift control of behaviour from one hemisphere to the other. Michael Gazzaniga, of Cornell University Medical College, still believes that in ordinary people the left brain is truly dominant. He finds the right hemisphere severely limited in its cognitive capacity.

The philosopher Roland Pucetti, of Canada's Dalhouise University, believes that the right hemisphere is so competent on its own that it constitutes a separate consciousness. He describes our two minds like two tap dancers performing in almost perfect unison, having qualitatively but not quantitatively the same experience.

Others such as neuropsychologists Elkhonon Goldberg, of the Albert Einstein College of Medicine and Louis Costa, of the University of Victoria, consider the right hemisphere to be the brain's jack of all trades. It's a generalist that addresses new problems without preconception and tries many solutions until it hits on one that works. The left hemisphere, in contrast, is a specialist, solving familiar problems quickly and efficiently by using established methods.

The right brain reflects on the left side of the body, and vice versa. In a balanced reading there will be no voltage showing on the voltmeter. In a reading where the right brain predominates, the voltage of the left hand will be higher than that of the right, so a positive reading will be seen. If the left brain is dominant, then the right hand will have a higher voltage than the left, and the reading will be in the negative range.

How can this help us? If the patient is calm and simply wants to discuss a problem, then the voltages will be around the zero. If the patient is suffering from anxiety, this shows more in the right brain than the left and the reading will be positive. If the person is left-brained, an intellectual, and a thinker as opposed to a feeler, the reading will be negative.

I am not implying that thinking states are negative states. It's just that the voltage of one brain is negative or positive with respect to the other part.

To try this yourself, obtain a good quality high impedance voltmeter with a large digital screen. Older types with needles are totally unsuitable. Attach to the leads two copper rods. Use the 0–200 Mv d.c. range. Test the conductivity of the rods and the efficiency of the connections by touching the rods together. The reading should be a steady zero. When the client has sat down, switch on the voltmeter and then ask them to hold the rods. Ensure that the positive terminal is in the left hand and the negative terminal is in the right hand. Make a careful note of the initial voltage and write it down. Make a series of observations over a test period which should not be less than one minute. Until you are used to the method, a good rule of thumb is to make observations once every ten seconds.

Here is an example of a reading:

Time (secs)	0	10	20	30	40	50	60
Voltage (mv)	+30	+20	+16	+14	+12	+5	+5

This person is initially nervous but settles down in preparation for the reading. Remember that a 'plus' reading indicates predominance of feeling over thinking.

However, in this next example, matters are more complicated:

Time (secs)	0	10	20	30	40	50	60
Voltage (mv)	+20	+4	−16	−8	−0	+5	+15

The brain activity is full of conflict and will be unable to think clearly and follow the gist of any thoughts that are put to it. One hemisphere is dominant followed by the other. Such a person will seldom hear what is being said to them.

In the third example, matters are apparently much more stable:

Time (secs)	0	10	20	30	40	50	60
Voltage (mv)	−4	−5	−3	−4	−5	−6	−5

This is a person who is 'stuck' mentally and who cannot feel emotional patterns. Such a person needs to be addressed very carefully and logically making sure that one point is understood before moving on to the next.

This final example is of a healer:

Time (secs)	0	10	20	30	40	50	60
Voltage (mv)	+2	+2	+1	+1	0	−1	−2

In this person the capacity for being a good counsellor is very much developed. It will take a lot to ruffle them. They are stable and reliable. They can see problems from both sides.

It is necessary for practitioners to make their own observations, and persevere until a pattern emerges. You will then discern almost instinctively what is right or wrong as a doctor with his stethoscope will know what is wrong with a patient.

CHECKING THE AURA AND ITS COMPONENTS

It is now time to examine the aura of the patient. This method has great advantages over conventional psychotherapy and counselling. It is based on the notion that the

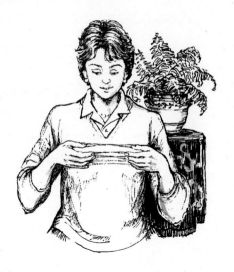

Learning to feel the auric radiations from your hands.

aura 'knows' what its needs are and is trying to convey this to the world around. When we speak of someone being 'needy' or 'confused' we are not so much talking about their conversation but what emanates from them. If you ask a person what is wrong with them, or what they need, they will report from the mind, which will include much social programing and will seldom encapsulate the real cause.

For example, a client might say that they are suffering from depression and they want to change their job. The real fact is that they have not recovered from a relationship break up, have no social life and blame their state on their job. To work through this may require four or five sessions with a counsellor with the consequent risk of waste of time and money. For effective and immediate work it is good to get to the nub of a problem right away. The client then knows that they cannot hide or defend themselves – and this is a great incentive for them to work!

Emanations happen from all parts of the body but in particular from the hands. The hands are notable for their unique signature in the fingerprints, the numerous acupuncture points and the formative and prophetic indications which some people lay store by in the form of palmistry. The hands radiate the equivalent of a bar code, the sort that is on every item of merchandise. How do we know that? Burr and Northrup, and the early radionic practitioners, discovered the existence of 'standing waves' which were detected by a high-impedence voltmeter. Although this was done in the 1930's, neither the work nor its implications have been followed through. The implications are significant – that the human body is surrounded by a lattice-work or grid of bioenergetic information. Since the DNA coding of each person is unique, it is reasonable to assume that the corresponding lattice-work is unique but, as they say, don't take my word for it!

First, here is an exercise which everyone can do, and is designed to tune you into these fields around your own body. This method is a preparation for working with a client, which is best done in the company of others, since for some reason the effect is greater.

Place your fingers about 9 inches apart facing each other. Move your hands towards each other and then slightly from side to side. Do not make any mental effort but merely concentrate on any sensations. You may feel prickles in the fingers of one or both hands. Notice how the prickles vary with the movement.

With a client the method is somewhat similar. Using the left hand on top and the right hand on the bottom, held about 9 inches apart, ask your client to put their left

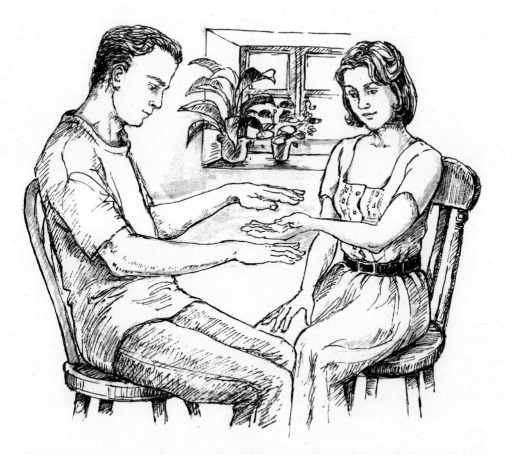

FEELING THE AURA OF THE OTHER PERSON. *Until you are used to this, the exercise should be carried out in a quiet environment. The practioner should move his left hand up and down until the sensation is maximized in their own hand. 'Mirror mode' can then take place involving the client reporting what he or she feels.*

hand between yours. Make sure that their hand is palm up and your hands palm down. Move your hands up and down until you feel a prickle in your own hand. Contact will then have been achieved.

There are two modes of doing this, both of which require a lot of practise. The first one is mirror mode. It requires you to programme your mind to bounce back these emanating bar codes to the client and for them to tell you what they feel. In other words, to use your hand as a mirror. This is particularly useful when demonstrating the method to a group, or when a third person is present. The second method is simply listening to the client's aura and obtaining a printout in your own hand as to what is going on.

Using either method, various reactions are obtained. These are heat, cold, heat alternating with cold, pressure, draughts, lines, prickles and sensations in other parts of the body. This is the aura's code for letting us know what is amiss, or what groups of tasks the person needs to do in order to take the next step on the road to development. In England we call it a 'queue', in America, a 'line'. Though some considerable experience is required to identify all the nuances, these are the meanings which will do as a start:

Heat – the need for emotional support

Cold – the ability to heal

Draught – the talent for working in a group; if combined with cold, to bring about healing

Prickles – the need to learn, to make sense of

Pressure – the need to resolve a relationship problem

Electric lines – the need for change in an aspect of your life

A reaction on the wrist – difficulties with birth and childhood

A reaction up the arm old material from previous lives

The areas in which the impressions happen are vital. In psychosomatic medicine (my speciality) the meanings of the fingers are the same as the interpretation of the Kirlian print as described in full in my book *The Unseen Self – Kirlian Photography Explained*.

Thumb – will power

Index finger – leadership ability

Middle finger – work/career situation

Fourth finger – creativity

Fifth finger – heart/spiritual matters

Electric lines at the side of the relevant fingers indicate a conflict between what a client is doing and what they would like to do.

Make a careful note of the order in which events happen. It is useful to have a chart with an outline of the hand for a third party to use to record the changes (where this is possible). When the client has reported their first impression, remove your hand and 'flick' it as if you were flicking off water. Then replace the hand and see if the impression or electrical print changes. If not, then the aura has but one message. For example, if the client reports cold, followed by more cold, then all they need to do is to develop their healing abilities. If repeating the experiment results in a change, then the aura has more than one immediate priority.

Therefore, the order in which the impressions happen are of key significance. A subject might get warmth followed by cold. This would mean that emotional support is required in order to encourage them to use their healing.

If this test is done methodically it will be an enormous benefit to the counselling and healing procedure.

DOWSING OR MEASURING OF THE ENERGY LEVELS

It is good practise to have three or four methods of diagnosis at one's disposal. I employ some dowsing methods using a pendulum. This is very good for the measurement of energy levels, though I believe it can result in over-stimulation of the chakras if you rely on the pendulum too much. Many dowsers find that they 'know'

first impression – warm in palm
second – line on index finger
third – warm on obverse
four – cold in palm
five – 'prick' at the end of middle finger
six – prickles at the end of all fingers

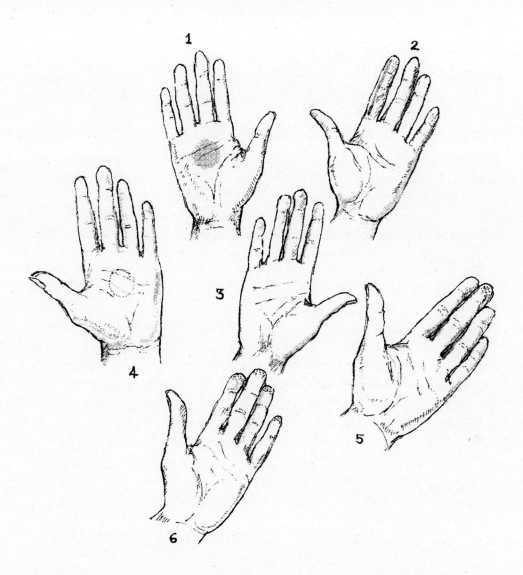

The aura has a 'queueing system' which announces its needs and priorities. Up to six different impressions can be gained from one experiment. When a sensation has been recieved, the practitioner should flick the left hand to remove the charge and then repeat. Take careful note of what happens.

even before picking up the pendulum what the answer to a problem might be. The eventual goal is to become free of all aids but with most of us this will take some time. To achieve these results you need to have had experience in dowsing. If you lack this experience, then use the second method described.

This part of the method works best with those with the mental discipline to programme their mind. Draw a graph with physical, mental, emotional and spiritual aspects delineated.

PHYSICAL

0–10	0	10	20	30	40	50	60	70	80	90	100

MENTAL

0–10	0	10	20	30	40	50	60	70	80	90	100

EMOTIONAL

0–10	0	10	20	30	40	50	60	70	80	90	100

SPIRITUAL

0–10	0	10	20	30	40	50	60	70	80	90	100

Using a pendulum, enquire mentally of your client the level of energy on the chosen field – say the mental side. Think up the numbers from one to one hundred. At that level the pendulum will change direction or orientation. Note the figure on the chart. Repeat for each of the other parameters. Even if one practitioner has a different understanding to another about the meaning of the word 'spiritual' or 'physical' you will refine this over time. I cannot emphasize the importance of practise and repetition. You will make the method your own.

If the pendulum does not work for you then try another method. Using the middle fingertip of your left hand (or right hand if that works better for you) ask the same mental question whilst running your finger from one end of the scale to the other. You will have programmed your mind to pick up the fields of the client and projected them on to a target where an interference pattern is formed. The human aura, with its ability to detect bioenergetic fields and standing waves, will react with a small shock and inform the practitioner. Reading this in cold print will cause a feeling of incredulity. The only comment I have is, "well, try it!".

This will then form the basis for you to use your professional skills to assist the client to face their problems. I have a shrewd suspicion that when a practitioner tunes into a problem they are also providing healing. Identifying a problem precisely seems to include within it the mechanism for release.

The meanings of the levels will be dealt with elsewhere, but through experience you will be able to understand where the stresses and strains are falling on an individual. Here are a few examples:-

Physical 70%;   Mental 50%;   Emotional 60%;   Spiritual 70%.

This is a near-ideal example. A variation of no more than 10% indicates a good degree of self-motivation and health.

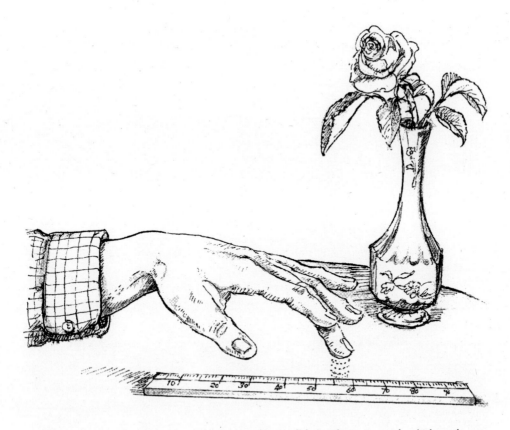

It is possible to use the hand as a dowsing instrument. Learn to 'listen' to slight impulses – no matter how irrelevant they may seem. Th best effect will be when the fingers are about 2 cm away from the rule or diagram

Physical 80%; Mental 30%; Emotional 50%; Spiritual 70%.

A person with general good health, under-stimulated at work; reasonably happy in their emotional life; a good faith in God from which they are sustained. The lowest reading is the weakest link in the chain so that is why it is good practise to pay attention to, in this case, the mental side. Ask them about mental stimulus, how well they are learning, whether they are bored with their job etc. 99% of the time, the reason for the dis-ease will emerge.

Physical 50%; Mental 60%; Emotional 1%; Spiritual 50%.

This is a client whose physical health is somewhat below the average, who has good mental functioning but who has had the bottom knocked out of their world by the breakdown of a relationship. Their spiritual level of 50% shows that they are having to re-think their beliefs and values.

Here the practitioner should commence with encouraging the client to talk about their past relationships. Frequently, people with good minds will say "oh no, that's all over now". That is merely the mind's attempt to heal the situation. The practitioners should indicate that they are aware of the seriousness of the situation and encourage the client to take it seriously. Such phrases as "the need to remove the last bit of pain" will encourage the client to work.

This analysis can be done within the first few minutes. Relying on reporting from the client could take ten times as long and thus more useful work can be achieved in a limited time.

DOWSING OR MEASURING THE CHAKRAS

Using the above methods, the seven major chakras can be measured. The ideal state is one of balance between them.

The summary meanings of the chakras are as follows

Crown	link with God, beliefs
Third eye	intuition, confidence
Throat	creativity
Heart	the ability to love others
Solar plexus	the energy derived from a partner or close associate
Sacral	sexual energy
Root	the link with the earth – practical matters – career choices.

Here is an example of a balanced set of chakras:-

```
Crown         open————————————x———————————closed
Third eye     open——————————————x—————————closed
Throat        open—————————x————————————————closed
Heart         open—————————x-————————————————closed
Solar plexus  open————————————x———————————closed
Sacral        open—————————x————————————————closed
Root          open—————————x————————————————closed
```

There is a slight deficiency of the third eye (intuition, confidence) and the solar plexus (relationships – caution) but this is balanced by the crown, heart and root which are centred.

Here is an example of an unbalanced set of chakras:-

```
Crown         open———————x—————————————————closed
Third eye     open————————————————x————————closed
Throat        open————————————————x————————closed
Heart         open————————x————————————————closed
Solar plexus  open———x———————x—————————x————closed
Sacral        open——————————————————————————closed
Root          open———————————————x—————————closed
```

This person lacks self confidence, is in a frustrating job, is insecure about their attractiveness, has damage in their solar plexus chakra through a counter-productive old relationship; suffered some child abuse (no reading on the sacral) and are lacking ambition in their job situation.

The combination of the energy readings and the chakra levels will give the practitioner a very good stereoscopic perspective on the whole matter and will then be able to assign a priority to the aspects of the personality that need to be addressed.

APPLYING HEALING

As many books on healing will have reminded you, we do not 'do' anything but enable the self-healing capacity of the living person with free will to assert itself. This is undoubtedly achieved not through what we practitioners say but through what we are. Healing means to draw out the poison, to resolve the conflict, to heal the wound. Healing, however, is only possible if we have a pure vibration ourselves. The impure cannot bring about purity. Nothing can happen unless the client permits it. Healing and listening are closely linked. It can take clients a long time to realize that they are being listened to, so unused are they to it. Many of my clients exhibit shock when I quote back at them what they said a few minutes previously.

At this point, the method of working is left to the individual practitioner.

HOW EFFECTIVE HAS THE SESSION BEEN?

Now is the time to establish if healing has taken place. This is done by checking aspects of the aura and of the energy field. There is one check that should normally be made.

VOLTMETER CHECK

We saw how the use of the voltmeter can establish the approximate nature of problem likely to be encountered. We can now use the same method to determine how effective the session has been. If there is no change, then there are two possibilities. The client does not want to get better or the practitioner is using the wrong method. This is a very accurate method of measuring the penetration value of the session.

Having said that, a message takes some time to be understood especially in those people who have had large blocks for some years. I recently saw a woman who had great difficulty remembering anything. She had been to see a great many specialists. I found that the memory problem was due to an early traumatic incident. She phoned up the day after saying that she could not understand the session. I asked her to listen to the tape that I always make during longer sessions. About a week passed. She then phoned up again, apologizing for her negative stance. She had listened to the tape five times, once with her husband, and now she understood what was being said. The shock of a diagnostic system that was different to normal allopathic medicine took some time to recover from!

Let's have a look at an example or two, using the figures quoted above of the unstable person. This was the reading prior to treatment. With an effective session you would hope to see a change.

Time (secs)	0	10	20	30	40	50	60
Voltage (mv)	+20	+4	−16	−8	−0	+5	+15

In this case the readings after were

Time (secs)	0	10	20	30	40	50	60
Voltage (mv)	+12	+10	+7	+3	−0	+1	+3

These would be very good results. They would mean that the client had accepted their situation and was prepared to work to improve themselves. Alas, in many cases there is not the desire to work and all the healing and listening in the world cannot get through that barrier.

If there is no change then the client should be asked if they feel comfortable with what has happened. There is ALWAYS a reason for no change. I would ask such a person to increase their commitment, and would probe to see if they had had an experience of unproductive professional attention.

This is only a fraction of what can be measured using the aura. To sum up, it is valuable because it saves time, promotes accuracy, involves the mind of the client because of its participatory nature and saves the time-consuming process of self-reporting which can lead to blind alleys. It also triggers many types of information such as images, ideas, words and even smells.

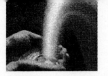

Chapter Fourteen

A REFLECTION ON FEAR

Socrates referred to an inner voice that guided him... "the prophetic voice to which I have become accustomed has always been my constant companion, opposing me even in quite trivial things if I was going to take the wrong course".

The action of speaking and of listening can function as a mysterious catalyst that unlocks material sometimes buried for years. But in addition to that, if we can more clearly understand the function of intuitive diagnosis as well as its sister art of healing, we can be more effective in our daily life. Such methods are non-invasive, safe, inexpensive and can cross boundaries which more conventional approaches do not start to do.

I recall seeing a man who had just been told by a psychiatrist that he needed treatment twice a week for two years as a treatment for depression. I examined and questioned him and found that he had strange feelings in his hands when certain people walked nearby. He also had strange visions. Had it occured to him, I asked, that he had budding psychic and sensitive abilities which were trying to assert themselves? Thunderstruck, he acknowledged that this might be the case. "That would fit" he mused when thinking of the symptoms. I asked him if he really wanted to see a psychiatrist. He replied that he did not see much point since no one had been able to help him in the past, but he simply did not know what else to do.

This case is typical of thousands of people but mercifully the 'New Age' trend of the 1970's is being maintained and is indeed maturing. The public is now looking with more favour on various forms of alternative and complementary medicine. The previous view was that impressions that do not come from a world of outer sense are dismissed as nonsense. Intuitive inspirations not derived from linear reasoning are deemed illogical. Some are now realizing that there is no one true picture of a patient's condition. Rather it is necessary to present one out of many possible pictures of reality. The medical, the spiritual and the psychological analyses should be super-imposed and an action taken from the whole to the part rather than treating a symptom often with drugs and hoping the whole system will restore its own equilibrium.

The problem is also one of language. Western healers are seldom medically trained and doctors have had scant time to work alongside healers and observe their methods. Such opportunities should not be missed. C. Norman Shealy, an

American surgeon who specializes in pain and stress management, found an intuitive diagnostician, Caroline Myss, who achieved a 93% diagnostic accuracy when given only the patient's name and birth date. By the same token, the reporting methodology of some psychics and practitioners leaves much to be desired. Science has given us a valuable legacy in the Scientific Method and people ignore this at their professional peril. I have found the book *The Art of Scientific Investigation* by W. I. B. Beveridge and *The Principles of Human Knowledge* by George Berkeley to be of great value in mustering the necessary discipline to bridge the gap between myself and my more conventional colleagues.

Another problem is that of fear. If people were offered a non- reversible drug that enabled them to detect the thoughts of everyone within a 100m radius, how many takers would there be? People often ask me if I can see the aura, and are quite disappointed when I reply that I can 'only feel' it. I am sure that if I were to have visual sightings of all the auras round me I would lose my mind in weeks!

I believe that the majority are more comfortable in their own constructed world, where they can decide on the parameters of truth. Do we want to be bothered with uncomfortable truth when it conflicts with years of habit? Jesus Christ summed it up when he said that "people who walk in darkness fear the light". The fact is that people only obtain a breakthrough when they decide, at whatever cost, to face themselves and their situation. That is where this book is designed to assist.

I hope these thoughts will have given readers some confidence to at least consider the value of intuition as an input to the problem solving process. No, everybody, it's not "just a thought". It is you using your intuition and picking up something that is not right. Listen – and save yourself a lot of pain.

I sometimes see clients in a specialist book shop, Mysteries, in central London. One day in the autumn of 1996, the owners informed me that some TV people were coming to film the shop. Would it be all right to use my material? I agreed. In due course, the camera crew arrived together with a scientist. Whilst they set up their equipment, the scientist paced around looking rather ill at ease. I sensed that they had come to do a 'hatchet job' as we say in the trade. Nevertheless I offered to show them my normal diagnostic method and said I would treat him the same as any other client. I remember joking with him that as this was a knocking programme, what I said or did would not make any difference – to which he made no comment.

I asked him to hold his hand between mine and to report on any feeling. "What do you feel?" I asked. "Nothing" said he. I adjusted my hands and asked him again. Again the reply was negative. "Well" I said "these experiments do not work 100% of the time." We concluded the session, apparently unsuccessfully.

Whilst the camera men were packing up, I happened to glance at the scientist out of the corner of my eye. There he was, large as life, looking very puzzled and flicking his hands as if trying to remove something. "Blow me down", I thought to myself, "He DID feel something". Of course he could not admit the fact to me because that would have undermined his hypothesis that there is nothing there. He was Prof.

Richard Dawkins, noted sceptic, and occupant of the Chair of Public Understanding of Science at Oxford University.

One of these fine days, I shall delight in reminding him of this story.

E-mail: consultant@pobox.com +44 (0) 181 670 4344
102 Thurlow Park Road, London SE21 8HY, UK

Brian Snellgrove is available for lectures, workshops, private consultations and healing. He travels widely and for work abroad needs to be contacted well in advance. Please E-mail or phone or write as convenient.

Chakra and Energy Analysis

completed for

_____

by

Brian Snellgrove

on

_____

England's leading

chakra analyst

Appointments and enquries - 0181 670 4344

E-mail consultant@pobox.com

Part one – *ENERGY-VITALITY LEVELS*

physical

_____|_____|_____

mental

_____|_____|_____

emotional

_____|_____|_____

spiritual

_____|_____|_____

Comments

Part two – RELATIONSHIPS PAST AND PRESENT

_____|_____|_____

_____|_____|_____

_____|_____|_____

_____|_____|_____

Comment and recommendation

Part three – OCCUPATION

_____|_____|_____

_____|_____|_____

Comment

Part four – CHAKRA ANALYSIS

A consultation gives you feedback on the overall condition of your aura, and of your chakras. The aura contains information about your situation past and present. We detect and measure the patterns.

First name _____ Marital status _____ Occupation. _____ Date _____

1st voltage reading from _____ To _____ Final reading from _____ To _____
A mark towards the *left* indicates an open chakra: to the *centre* a balanced chakra; to the *right* a closed chakra.

The CROWN chakra is your connection with your higher self. An open chakra does not necessarily mean that you are 'religious'. It indicates that higher forces are influencing your life – whether you are aware of it or not! It can be seen as an 'inner guidance' system and gives strength when we need it.

The AJNA chakra measures your intution through what is called the third eye. Some say that the soul resides in the pineal gland, which is midway between the eyes.

The THROAT is an indication of your creativity not just in your work but in your life in general. A closed reading means that your potential is not being realised.

The HEART measures how you are relating to everyone. We speak of people having a 'big heart'. Well, that's what this reading is all about! This is about the intimate and personal aspects of your being.

The SOLAR PLEXUS chakra contains an energy link between you, and the people to whom you have or have had a close connection. Often, disharmonious energies are transmitted through this chakra if a relationship ended unpleasantly.

The SACRAL chakra is connected with sexual energy. It is not about sexual encounters as such but the ability or wish to exchange intimacy.

The ROOT chakra is about our ability to function in the physical world; the ambition to survive.

Key words and comments

Hand reactions

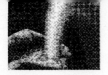

INDEX